SENESCENCE AND SENESCENCE-RELATED DISORDERS

Edited by **Zhiwei Wang**
and **Hiroyuki Inuzuka**

Senescence and Senescence-Related Disorders
http://dx.doi.org/10.5772/56158
Edited by Zhiwei Wang and Hiroyuki Inuzuka

Contributors

Patrizia D'Alessio, Kin-Ya Kubo, Sebastian Haferkamp, Therese Becker, David Bernard, Arnaud Augert, Ulrike Zentgraf, Stefan Bieker, Shavali Shaik

Published by InTech

Janeza Trdine 9, 51000 Rijeka, Croatia

Publishing Process Manager Danijela Duric
Technical Editor InTech DTP team
Cover InTech Design team

Additional hard copies can be obtained from orders@intechopen.com

Senescence and Senescence-Related Disorders, Edited by Zhiwei Wang and Hiroyuki Inuzuka
p. cm.
ISBN 978-953-51-0997-6

Meet the editors

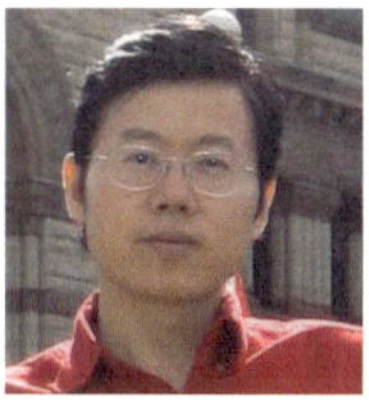

Dr. Zhiwei Wang is a professor in Cyrus Tang Hematology Center, Soochow University, P.R. China. He received his MD from Anhui Bengbu Medical College, P.R. China, and his Ph.D. from the Wayne State University, Michigan, USA. He has completed postdoctoral fellowships at Karmanos Cancer Institute, Wayne State University, Michigan, USA. Then, he was an instructor in Beth Israel Deaconess Medical Center, Harvard medical School, USA. He has published more than 140 papers in peer-reviewed journals with Hirsh Factor 31, and citations more than 3000. He has served as an ad hoc reviewer of grant and as an ad hoc reviewer of papers for more than 40 Journals. Dr. Wang's research interests are focused on the roles of cell signaling pathways such as Notch, FoxM1 and E3 ubiquitin ligases in senescence and tumorigenesis. Moreover, He is also interested in roles of microRNA and stem cells in drug resistance.

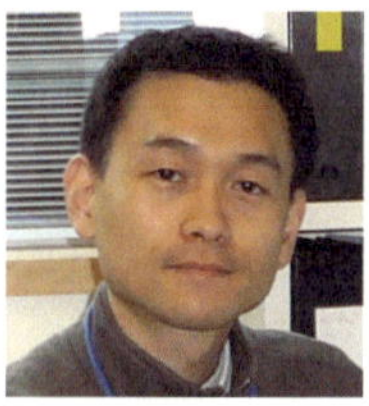

Dr. Hiroyuki Inuzuka is an instructor at Beth Israel Deaconess Medical Center and Harvard Medical School. He earned his Ph.D. in molecular biology from the University of Tokyo. His current research focuses on the molecular mechanisms of human malignancy including age-related diseases. Specifically, his studies involve uncovering the molecular processes involved in cell cycle regulation and cellular senescence. Ultimately, he seeks to apply his findings to help find a way to extend human healthy life expectancy.

Contents

Preface

This book discusses in detail regarding senescence and its related diseases. Each chapter is written by distinguished researchers and practicing clinicians, which provides unique, individual knowledge based on the expertise of the authors. This book should build further the endeavors of the readers in senescence field. Therefore, I wish that this book would serve as a basis for further discussions and developments in exploring molecular mechanism of senescence.

The first chapter, written by Dr. Shavali Shaik and his colleagues from Beth Israel Deaconess Medical Center Harvard Medical School, describes the molecular changes that occur in the vascular system due to aging, and defines how age-induced changes in the endothelium ultimately lead to the development of various vascular diseases. Dr. Shaik et al. highlighted particularly how the age-induced oxidative stress plays a major role in causing loss of endothelial function, and described the underlying mechanisms responsible for the development of various vascular diseases including cardiovascular, peripheral vascular and diabetic retinopathy which are highly observed in aged population.

The second chapter in this book, Dr. Becker Therese and colleagues provide detailed insight into the molecular mechanisms of how the two tumor suppressor pathways, p53-p21 and the p16INK4a-pRb, regulate the onset and maintenance of cellular senescence. They furthermore explain the molecular network regulating chromatin remodeling and the formation of senescence associated heterochromatin foci, with emphasis on the above mentioned pathways.

In the next chapter, Dr. Stefan Bieker et al. give an overview on the current knowledge on regulatory mechanisms of senescence in general and their impact on nitrogen metabolism, including uptake, assimilation, and distribution within the plant. Special attention was also given to reactive nitrogen and reactive oxygen molecules as signalling components in this complex regulatory network.

In the following chapter, Dr. David Bernard et al. introduce features, markers, triggers and molecular regulators of cellular senescence and discuss their role in tumorigenesis. Moreover, Dr. Bernard describes the role of immunosenescence in the development of cancer, suggesting that senescence immunosurveillance is pivotal for tumor eradication.

The next chapter, by Dr. Kubo Kin-ya et al., tries to provide evidence supporting the interaction between mastication and learning and memory. Dr. Kubo et al. briefly describe recent progress in understanding how mastication affects learning and memory. Moreover, they highlight the impaired function and pathology of the hippocampus in an animal model of reduced mastication. More importantly, they discuss how occlusal disharmony is a chronic stressor that suppresses hippocampal-mediated learning and memory.

The last chapter is by Dr. Claudio Franceschi and colleagues. They describe how to combat neurodegenerative disease using results obtained with ad hoc models such as centenarians and their offspring compared with subjects affected by Down syndrome. They also discuss future perspectives on the reversibility of early stages of degenerative diseases by non anti-inflammatory approaches including physical exercise, motivational implementation, nutrition and nutraceutic approaches. Importantly, they conclude the development of novel tools to be integrated in daily life of elderly people which is critical for reducing degenerative diseases.

Lastly, as the editors, we are grateful to the contributors for their promptness in preparing their chapters. We are also impressed by their dedication and diligent work. We are thankful to Dr. Wenyi Wei for strong support during publishing this book. We also appreciate receiving help from Ms. Danijela Duric.

Zhiwei Wang, Ph.D M.D
Harvard Medical School
Department of Pathology
Beth Israel Deaconess Medical Center
Boston, USA

Hiroyuki Inuzuka, PhD
Harvard Medical School
Department of Pathology
Beth Israel Deaconess Medical Center
Boston, USA

Section 1

Aging and Vascular Diseases

Chapter 1

Endothelium Aging and Vascular Diseases

Shavali Shaik, Zhiwei Wang, Hiroyuki Inuzuka,
Pengda Liu and Wenyi Wei

Additional information is available at the end of the chapter

http://dx.doi.org/10.5772/53065

1. Introduction

Aging is a biological process that causes a progressive deterioration of structure and function of all organs over the time [1]. According to the United Nation's report, the number of people aged 60 and over in the world has increased from 8% (200 million) in 1950 to 11% (760 million) in 2005, and it is estimated that this number will further increase to 22% (2 billion) in 2050. It is expected that in the US alone, the aged population of 65 and over will grow rapidly and reach 81 million by 2050 [2,3]. This rapidly increasing aging population will not only cause a decline of productive workforce but also negatively affect the country's economy. Furthermore, aging is one of the major risk factors for the development of many diseases including cardiovascular diseases [4], stroke [5] and cancer [6]. Moreover, the epidemiological data strongly suggests that more often these diseases are diagnosed in older people compared to younger individuals. In addition to the huge economical impact, these diseases also cause loss of productivity and disability in the elderly population. Therefore, it is extremely important to give high priorities to aging and age-associated disease research in order to develop novel therapies to slow the aging process as well as to prevent and /or treat the age-associated diseases more effectively. It has been found that many factors including genetics [7,8], metabolism [9], diet [10] and stress [11] can in part contribute to the aging process. Similar to other organs, the vascular system, which provides oxygen and nutrients to all the organs in the body, is also affected by the aging process and becomes more vulnerable to disease development in the elders [12,13]. For example, vascular diseases such as coronary artery disease, peripheral arterial disease, stroke and microvascular disease are more often found in the aged population. This is in part due to the structural and functional changes that occur in the vascular system of aged people. In this review, we highlighted (i) the changes that occur in the vascular system, particularly in the endothelium due to aging; (ii) the mechanisms by which the age-associated changes lead to decreased angiogenesis;

(iii) how the ubiquitin proteasome system plays important roles in regulating vascular endothelium function; (iv) the mechanisms by which the age-associated increase in oxidative stress might cause endothelial dysfunction; and finally, (iv) how the age-associated changes in the vascular system lead to the development of various vascular diseases such as coronary artery disease, peripheral artery disease and diabetic retinopathy.

2. Age-associated changes in the vascular system

Many changes are known to occur due to aging in the entire vascular system that includes heart, coronary arteries, peripheral arteries and small blood vessels known as capillaries (Figure 1). There will be an increase in the overall size of the heart, due to an increase in the heart wall thickness in the aging heart. The heart valves, which control the unidirectional of blood flow, will also become stiffer. There is also deposition of the pigments known as lipofuscin in the aged heart along with possible loss of cardiomyocytes as well as cells present in the sinoatrial node (SA node). Furthermore, there is an increase in the size of cardiomyocytes to compensate for the loss of the heart cells. These changes altogether cause a progressive decline in the physiological functions of the heart in the elderly population. In addition to these changes in the heart, the blood vessels also undergo significant changes. For example, the aorta, the large artery that originates from the heart becomes thicker, stiffer and less flexible. Smaller blood vessels also become thicker and stiffer. These changes are due to alterations that occur in the cells present in the blood vessels and also in the connective tissue of the blood vessel wall. All these changes ultimately lead to hypertrophy of the heart and causes an increase in the blood pressure [14]. There seems to be an interconnection between changes in the blood vessels and changes in the heart. Changes such as thickening of the blood vessels lead to increase in the blood pressure, which further affects the heart function. In that condition, the heart tries to function more efficiently by becoming larger in size (hypertrophy) and by enhancing its pumping capacity.

3. Changes that occur in the vascular endothelium

The vascular endothelium is comprised of a layer of endothelial cells that are positioned in the inner surface of blood vessels. The endothelium forms an interface between circulating blood and vessel wall, hence has a direct contact with circulating blood. In addition to serving as a barrier, endothelial cells participate in many physiological functions. They control vascular homeostasis, regulate blood pressure by vasoconstriction and vasodilatory mechanisms and promote angiogenesis when body requires. They also secrete anti-coagulatory factors to prevent clotting [15]. Importantly, vascular endothelial cells express many important molecules such as vascular endothelial growth factor (VEGF) and its receptors vascular endothelial growth factor receptor-1 (VEGFR1), vascular endothelial growth factor receptor-2 (VEGFR2) and vascular endothelial growth factor receptor-3 (VEGFR3). VEGFR1 and VEGFR2 are expressed exclusively in vascular endothelial cells, whereas VEGFR3 is mainly

http://dx.doi.org/10.5772/53065

expressed in the lymphatic endothelial cells [16]. The VEGF/VEGFR2 signaling is critical for vasculogenesis as well as angiogenesis [16]. Disruption or loss of VEGF and VEGFR2 genes is associated with severe vascular abnormalities or embryonic lethality [17]. Furthermore, the endothelial cells produce other growth factors known as angiopoitins (Ang), which are required to remodel and stabilize the immature blood vessels induced by VEGF/VEGFR2. Moreover, molecules such as neuropilines are involved in modulating the binding as well as responses to VEGF receptors [16]. Furthermore, endothelial cells express endothelial nitric oxide synthase (eNOS), which produces nitric oxide (NO). NO has many important physiological functions. For example, NO promotes vasodilation [18], as well as inhibits leukocyte adhesion [19], thrombocyte aggregation [20] and smooth muscle cell proliferation [21]. Under basal conditions eNOS is found inactive, however its activity is increased by many factors including acetyl choline, bradykinin, thrombin and histamine that lead to increased production of NO.

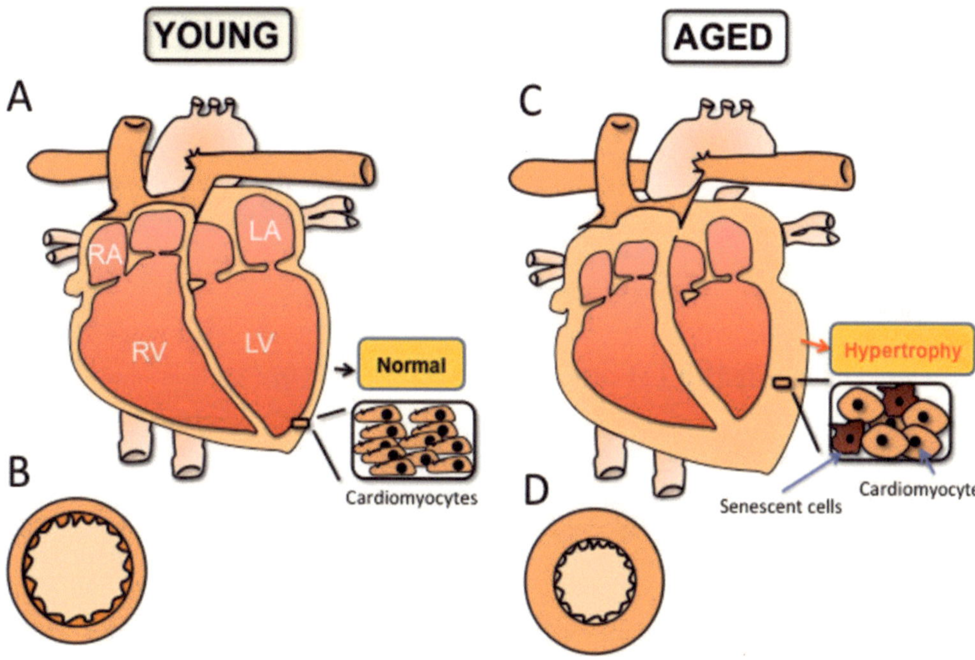

Figure 1. Age-associated changes that occur in the heart and the vascular system. Normal young heart has highly functional cardiomyocytes, and normal atrium and ventricles (A). Young artery has normal lumen, normal arterial thickness and efficient contractile and relaxation properties (B). However, aged heart has increased thickness in the heart muscle due to hypertrophy. Specifically, cardiomyocytes from aged heart show hyperplasia along with some cardiomyocytes undergoing senescence (C). Aged artery also has increased thickness, reduced lumen and less efficient contractile and relaxation properties (D). These age-associated changes ultimately lead to reduced cardiac as well as vascular functions in the elders.

Aging also influences endothelial cells and causes a progressive deterioration of their function. Previous studies have shown that endothelium-mediated vasodilatory function progressively declines with age [22]. This is associated with decreases in eNOS expression and NO production by aging endothelial cells [23,24]. Recently, Yoon et al. have shown that decreased expression of eNOS in aged human umblical vein endothelial cells [24]. However, the precise mechanisms for the age-associated decreases of these molecules remain unknown. Interestingly, it has been observed that the aging endothelial cells produce increased amount of O_2-anions [25], which scavenge NO to form peroxinitrite, a potent form of free radical. Peroxinitrite further inactivates eNOS and decreases its activity [26]. These described mechansims in part explain oxidative stress-mediated decrease of eNOS and NO in aging endothelial cells. On the other hand, it has been suggested that the age-associated changes that occur in eNOS regulatory proteins such as caveolin-1, pAkt, and heat shock protein 90 (Hsp90) contribute to the decreased activity of eNOS in aged endothelial cells [24]. In addition to these regulatory mechanisms, several other factors also regulate eNOS activity. For example, shear stress [27], estrogens [28], and growth factors [29] could also positively regulate eNOS expression. However, as their expression levels decrease with advancing in age, these changes might cause a subsequent decrease in eNOS expression. Taken together, these alterations finally lead to both a decreased expression of eNOS and decreased levels of NO in aged endothelial cells. In addition to these changes in endothelial cells, aging also causes several other changes in vascular smooth muscle cells (VSMCs). During the aging process, VSMCs migrate from tunica media to tunica intima and start accumulating there. These cells become less functional and less responsive to growth factors such as transforming growth factor-beta1 [30]. As VSMCs are important regulatory cells that control the vascular wall by vasoconstriction and vasodilatory mechanisms, progressive loss of their physiological functions might lead to changes in vascular endothelium and impaired vascular function in the aged blood vessels.

4. Aging causes impaired angiogenesis

Angiogenesis, the formation of new blood vessels from pre-existing vessels, is a physiologically an important process during growth, menstrual cycle and wound healing. Several factors are known to influence angiogenesis. The most important one is hypoxia, which activates the transcription factors such as hypoxia-inducible factor-1 alpha (HIF-1 alpha) and peroxisome proliferator-activated receptor gamma coactivator-1 alpha (PGC-1 alpha) [31]. These transcription factors increase the production of VEGF and other growth factors that promote proliferation and migration of vascular endothelial cells. During angiogenesis, matrix metalloproteinases, the enzymes that degrade the capillary basement membrane and extra-cellular matrix, will be increased in order to facilitate endothelial cell migration. Therefore, angiogenesis is a complex process, and its timely induction is tightly controlled by coordination from multiple factors. Unfortunately, angiogenesis is markedly reduced by aging [32]. In keeping with this notion, wound healing, which is associated with angiogenesis, is also markedly impaired in aged mice [33] and significantly delayed and impaired in aged individuals [34]. Several studies were attempted to find the age-associated changes that might cause impaired angiogenesis. To this end, it has been observed that aging endothelial cells are functionally less angiogenic and less responsive to growth factors [32]. Rivard et al. [32] have found that VEGF levels were markedly reduced in aging mice. During hind limb ischemia, the old mice are unable to produce sufficient VEGF levels compared to younger mice, which are critically necessary for neovascularization and proper wound healing. Furthermore, the T lymphocyte-derived VEGF also markedly reduced in old mice, which compromised the angiogenesis-mediated wound healing process during the hind limb ischemia. This study, therefore, identified loss of VEGF as one of the key factors for the impaired angiogenesis observed in aged mice [32]. Furthermore, Qian et al. found that in addition to VEGF decrease, its key receptor VEGFR2 levels were also significantly decreased in eNOS knockout old mice [35]. Since the VEGF/VEGFR2 signaling is crucial for the survival, proliferation and migration of endothelial cells, a decrease of this pivotal signaling pathway may lead to impaired angiogenesis and delayed wound healing in aged subjects. Even in the eNOS knockout mice, which produce significantly less NO, the angiogenic response was markedly less in older mice due to decreased expression of VEGFR2. This partially explains that VEGFR2 plays an important role in neovascularization even in the absence of eNOS and corresponding NO [35].

Importantly, in addition to the loss of pro-angiogenic molecules, the anti-angiogenic molecules such as thrombospondin-2 (TSP2) levels were also affected by aging. To demonstrate the significance of TSP2 in aging and wound healing process, Agah et al. created full thickness excisional wounds in TSP2 null young and TSP2 null old mice and observed the wound healing process [36]. Consistent with other groups [33], they found that regardless of TSP genetic status, the would healing is delayed in old mice in comparison with young mice. However, interestingly, they found that the wound healing was faster in TSP2 null, old mice compared to wild-type, old mice suggesting that increased TSP2 in older mice might delay the angiogenesis and wound healing process. Correspondingly, there was also impaired expression of matrix metalloproteinase-2 (MMP2) found in TSP2 null old mice. These age-associated increase in expression of TSP2 and impaired MMP2 expression in older mice together might cause impaired angiogenesis and delay the wound healing process [36]. In addition to these changes observed in older mice, there are also changes observed in cell cycle-related molecules, which may affect the proliferation of aged endothelial cells. For example, aged endothelial cells undergo senescence and cease proliferation, which may limit neovascularization. Indeed, after certain passages, human umbilical vein endothelial cells (HUVECs) known to undergo senescence and loose their proliferative capacity [37]. As NO is known to prevent endothelial cell senescence, age associated decreases in eNOS and NO may be in part responsible for the senescence observed in HUVECs. Interestingly, the telomerase reverse transcriptase (TERT), which prevents senescence by counteracting telomere shortening process is active in human endothelial cells. However, after several passages, endothelial cells display a decrease of NO and loss of TERT activity that further lead to endothelial senescence. Indeed, ectopic overexpression of TERT protects from endothelial cells from undergoing senescence and preserve the angiogenic function of endothelial cells [38]. Furthermore, TERT overexpression increased eNOS function and enhanced precursor endothelial cell proliferation and migration that effectively promoted angiogenesis [39,40]. In fact, TERT expression decreased p16 and p21 activities that are significantly increased in senescent endothelial cells. These findings indicate that loss of telomerase-induced senescence also plays a role in affecting angiogenesis in aged endothelial cells. Interestingly, in a separate set of experiments, it has been demonstrated that VEGF-A, a potent pro-angiogenic factor, suppresses both p16 and p21 activities in endothelial cells, suggesting that VEGF-A could serve as an anti-senescence agent [41]. However, it remains unclear whether VEGF-A activates the VEGFR2 kinase to influence hTERT activity to exert this anti-senescence capacity. Taken together, these findings indicate that even though there is a shift between pro-angiogenic and anti-angiogenic molecules in aged endothelial cells, it remains to be determined whether increasing pro-angiogenic factors or inhibiting anti-angiogenic molecules restores angiogenesis and accelerate wound healing process especially by aged endothelial cells. Future research are therefore warranted to thoroughly address these important questions.

5. Aging-induced oxidative stress and vascular endothelial dysfunction

Oxidative stress is implicated in causing aging of endothelium and endothelial dysfunctions. In turn, aged endothelium produces increased free radicals, which might further accelerates aging. Based upon biomarkers of oxidant damage, increased levels of nitrotyrosine were observed in human aged vascular endothelial cells [42], Moreover, oxidative stress markers were also observed in the arteries of aged animals [26,43], suggesting that aging is indeed associated with increased formation of reactive oxygen species (ROS). Many different mechanisms are responsible for causing oxidative stress in endothelial cells that includes mitochondria-mediated production of ROS, decreases in free radical scavengers and increased susceptibility of macromolecules to free radical damage. Similar to other cells, oxidative stress damages proteins, lipids and DNA in vascular endothelial cells, thus causing loss of endothelial cell function. One of the major free radicals is super oxide anion (O_2^-), which is produced by aging mitochondria due to increased mitochondrial DNA damage. It has been demonstrated that NADPH contributes to O_2^- generation in vascular endothelial cells. Usually, the O_2^- anions are detoxified to H_2O_2 by manganese super oxide dismutase (MnSOD), which is present in the mitochondria. However, in the presence of NO, O_2^- leads to formation of a potent free radical known as peroxinitrite ($ONOO^-$) that further damages macromolecules in the endothelial cells. It has been demonstrated that $ONOO^-$ can inactivate both MnSOD and eNOS in the endothelial cells [44]. The switch of eNOS from an NO generating enzyme to an O_2^- generating enzyme (NO synthase uncoupling) leads to increased production of O_2^- and enhanced oxidative stress in aged endothelial cells (Figure 2). Taken together, NADPH and eNOS are important contributors for O_2^- generation in aged endothelial cells, since inhibition of NADPH and eNOS attenuates O_2^- production in the aorta of aged Wistar-Kyoto rats [25].

http://dx.doi.org/10.5772/53065

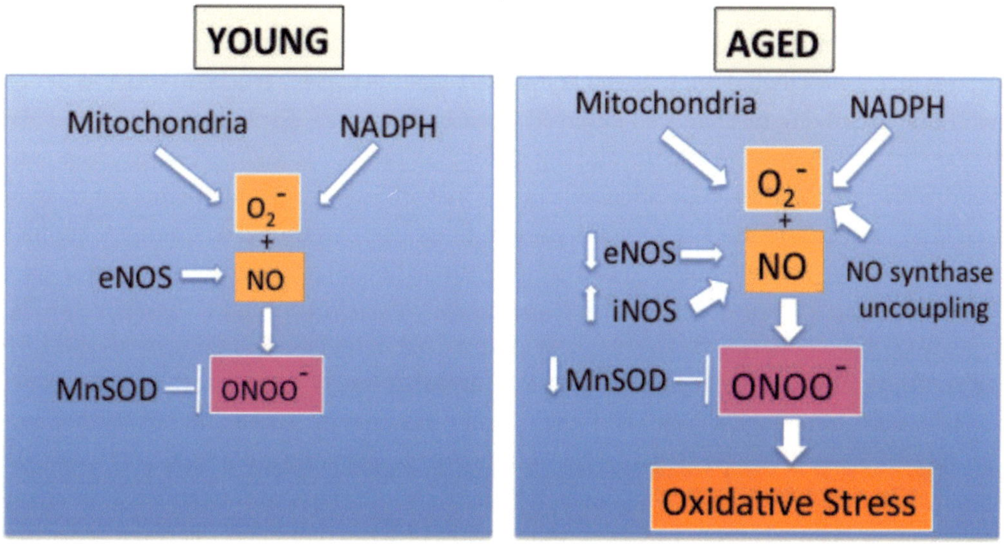

Figure 2. Oxidative stress in aged endothelial cells. Compared to younger endothelial cells, aged endothelial cells produce increased levels of free radicals. In the presence of nitric oxide (NO), which is originated from iNOS in aged endothelial cells, O_2^- lead to formation of a potent free radical known as peroxinitrite ($ONOO^-$). These changes lead to increased oxidative stress that damages macromolecules and ultimately lead to loss of endothelial cell function in aged cells.

The potential role of oxidative stress in vascular endothelium aging is also evident from the experiments carried out with antioxidants. For example, Vitamin C has been shown to decrease telomere shortening and increase the longevity of endothelial cells in culture [45]. N-Acetylcysteine, a potent antioxidant known to decrease endothelial cell senescence by preserving TERT activity and preventing its nuclear export [46]. Interestingly, it has been demonstrated that p66shc deletion protects endothelial cells from aging-associated vascular dysfunction [43] and sirtuins decrease the p66shc expression [47]. Although human clinical trials with antioxidants such as Vitamin C and E have not yielded beneficial effects on improving cardiovascular function [48,49], future studies with other antioxidants such as N-acetylcysteine may yield positive results in improving endothelial dysfunction associated with aging and oxidative stress.

6. Ubiquitin-proteasome system regulates endothelial cell function

The ubiquitin-proteasome system (UPS) plays important roles in a variety of key cellular functions including cellular protein homeostasis, signal transduction, cell cycle control, immune function, cellular senescence and apoptosis. This system targets specific proteins in the cell for degradation via ubiquitination-mediated destruction mechanism by specific ubiquitin E3 ligases [50,51]. Two major complexes, Skp1-Cul-1-F-box protein complex (SCF) and Anaphase Promoting Complex/Cyclosome (APC/C) are involved in the regulation of cell cycle as well as other key regulatory processes in the cell. Dysfunction of UPS leads to development of many diseases including cancer and cardiovascular disease. Therefore, how UPS regulates endothelial cell function and endothelial cell cycle is crucial in order to understand the underlying mechanisms involved in vascular disease development, and will also provide important insights into developing novel therapies for many vascular diseases associated with aging. Increasing evidence suggests that UPS regulates endothelial function by specifically regulating the key proteins present in endothelial cells. For example, the half-lives of both eNOS and inducible nitric oxide synthase (iNOS) are regulated by proteasome-dependent degradation [52,53]. Furthermore, the von Hippel-Lindau protein (pVHL) regulates HIF-1 alpha, which is a critical factor involved in regulating angiogenesis [54] (Figure 3). Consistent with the key role of UPS in endothelial function, treatment with low doses of proteasome inhibitor increases endothelial cell function [55]. These findings further suggest that UPS could be a potential target to improve the physiological functions of vasculature, hence may be utilized as a valuable drug target to develop novel treatments for aging-associated vascular diseases. However, the specific E3 ligase complexes and the molecular mechanisms that are involved in the regulation of endothelial cell cycle and endothelial cell function remain unknown.

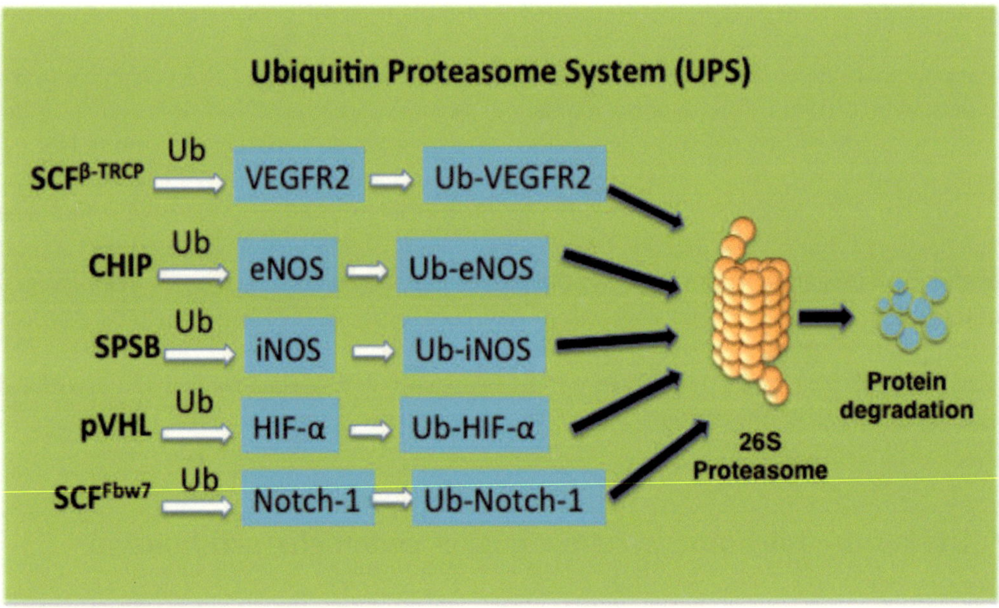

Figure 3. The ubiquitin proteasome system (UPS) regulates the stability of various key proteins in endothelial cells. The E3 ubiquitin ligases such as SCF$^{\beta\text{-TRCP}}$, C-terminus of Hsp70-interacting protein (CHIP), SOCS box-containing protein [ECS(SPSB)] and pVHL, target VEGFR2, eNOS, iNOS and HIF-1 alpha, respectively, for proteasome-dependent degradation. These E3 ligases recognize their respective substrates once the substrates are properly phosphorylated at the critical phosphodegrons by one or more kinases. This is an important regulatory mechanism by which UPS controls the half-lives of various key proteins in endothelial cells to influence the angiogenesis process.

Recent studies indicate that F-box proteins such as SCF^{Fbw7} and $SCF^{\beta\text{-}TRCP}$ are potentially involved in regulating endothelial cell function. For example, mice lacking Fbw7 die early (embryonic day 10.5) with developmental defects in vascular and haematopoietic system as well as heart chamber maturation [56,57]. As Fbw7 regulates the key cell cycle regulators including Notch, cyclin E, c-Myc and c-Jun, deletion of Fbw7 leads to accumulation of these substrates in the endothelial and /or hematopoitic cells. Indeed, elevated Notch protein levels were observed in Fbw7-deficient embryos that lead to the deregulation of the transcriptional repressor, Hey1, which is an important factor for cardiovascular development [56]. Therefore, these findings suggest that Fbw7 is an important E3 ligase governing the timely destruction of the key substrates involved in cardiovascular development. Furthermore, our laboratory has recently identified $SCF^{\beta\text{-}TRCP}$ as an E3 ubiquitin ligase that is potentially involved in regulating VEGFR2 protein levels in microvascular endothelial cells [58]. As stated in above sections, VEGFR2 is the major regulator of angiogenesis. Increased angiogenesis is associated with certain cancers, whereas angiogenesis is markedly decreased in aging individuals. Our study, for the first time, revealed that deregulation of β-TRCP leads to stabilization of VEGFR2 and subsequent increases in angiogenesis, whereas increased β-TRCP activity leads to decreased VEGFR2 levels and reduced angiogenesis. Mechanistically, casein kinase-I (CKI)-induced phosphorylation of VEGFR2 at critical phospho-degrons leads to its ubiquitination by β-TRCP, and subsequent degradation of VEGFR2 through the 26S proteasome [58]. However, we are just beginning to understand the critical role of UPS in endothelial function, future studies are therefore warranted to unravel the important role of various E3 ubiquitin ligases in the regulation of vascular system, which may ultimately, help to prevent vascular diseases in the elderly population.

7. Aging and vascular diseases

Aging vascular endothelium is susceptible to the development of various vascular diseases including cardiovascular disease (CVD) (coronary artery disease; atherosclerosis and hypertension), peripheral vascular disease (PVD), diabetic retinopathy, renal vascular disease and micro-vascular disease. Importantly, aging-associated changes that occur in the blood vessels are the major cause for the development of these diseases. Therefore, identifying the molecular changes that occur in the aging-endothelium and elucidating the underlying molecular mechanisms responsible for vascular disease development lead to the development of novel therapies to treat various vascular diseases.

7.1. Cardiovascular and peripheral vascular diseases

Cardiovascular disease (CVD) is the number one cause of human death in the US as well as in the world. CVD mostly occur in the aged population [59], and according to the World Health Organization, an estimated 17.3 million deaths occurred due to CVD in 2008. Coronary artery disease (CAD) is the major form of CVD, which occurs when coronary arteries are blocked due to atherosclerosis. Aging endothelium is very susceptible for plaque formation that leads to progressive blockage of the coronary arteries. This causes reduced blood supply (decreased supply of oxygen and nutrients) to the affected area of the heart. Although partial blockages may cause symptoms such as angina, complete loss of blood supply leads to heart attack, and if not treated immediately, may lead to sudden death. It has been observed that several age-associated changes in the endothelium-derived factors are responsible for plaque formation in the arteries. Importantly, endothelin (ET), a vascular endothelium-derived growth factor was found to be significantly increased in the aged endothelium [60,61,62]. ET mainly acts through its receptors ET-A and ET-B present on endothelial as well as vascular smooth muscle cells (VSMCs). ET-A activation leads to the constriction and proliferation of VSMCs, whereas ET-B activation leads to increased production of NO, which leads to vasodilation and inhibition of platelet aggregation. Studies indicate that ET-A receptor is mainly involved in the development of atherosclerosis, as inhibition of ET-A receptor prevents atherosclerosis in apolipoprotein-E deficient mice [63]. More importantly, endothelin-1 also decreases eNOS in vascular endothelial cells through ET-A receptor activation [64], suggesting that aging-induced increases in ET-1 as well as increased activation of ET-A receptor are potentially involved in causing atherosclerosis. Furthermore, the aging-induced increased expression of various adhesion molecules, such as intercellular adhesion molecule-1 (ICAM-1) and vascular cell adhesion molecule-1 (VCAM-1) also contribute to the ongoing process of atherosclerosis [65].

Inflammation, another major factor that is also known to increase with aging potentially contribute to the process of atherosclerosis [66]. Consistently, the incidence of atherosclerosis is found much higher in patients with autoimmune diseases such as rheumatoid arthritis [67,68] and systemic lupus erythematosus [69]. Several different immune cells and increased expression of adhesion molecules also play a major role in developing atherosclerotic plaque. For instance, adhesion molecules ICAM-1 and VCAM-1 not only facilitate the binding of immune cells such as monocytes and T-cells, but also help to transport these cells into the arterial wall. Once inside, the monocytes differentiate into macrophages, and ultimately become foam cells by taking up the oxidized LDL. The proteoglycans present in the extra cellular space of the intima bind with the oxidized LDL molecules. Moreover, the activated T-cells secrete several different cytokines that promote inflammation and activate VSMCs to proliferate. Altogether, this ongoing inflammatory process accelerates the process of atherosclerosis and damages the coronary arterial wall [70] (Figure 4).

Atherosclerosis is also occurs in other arteries other than coronary arteries. If atherosclerosis occurs in the peripheral arteries then it is called peripheral vascular disease or peripheral arterial disease (PAD). PAD is also influenced by aging and mostly occurs in elderly population. The prevalence increases with age from 3% under 60 years of age to 20% in aged 70 years and over [71]. Several factors influence the development of PAD that includes smoking, dyslipidemia, hypertension, diabetes and platelet aggregation. Advanced atherosclerosis in coronary arteries leads to angina and heart attack, whereas in cerebral arteries leads to stroke or transient ischemic attacks. If atherosclerosis occurs in peripheral arteries, that will lead to pain during walking or exercising (claudication), and this condition causes defects in the wound healing or ulcers. Preventing or slowing down the age-associated changes that occurs in the vascular system will protect the aged population from developing various vascular diseases.

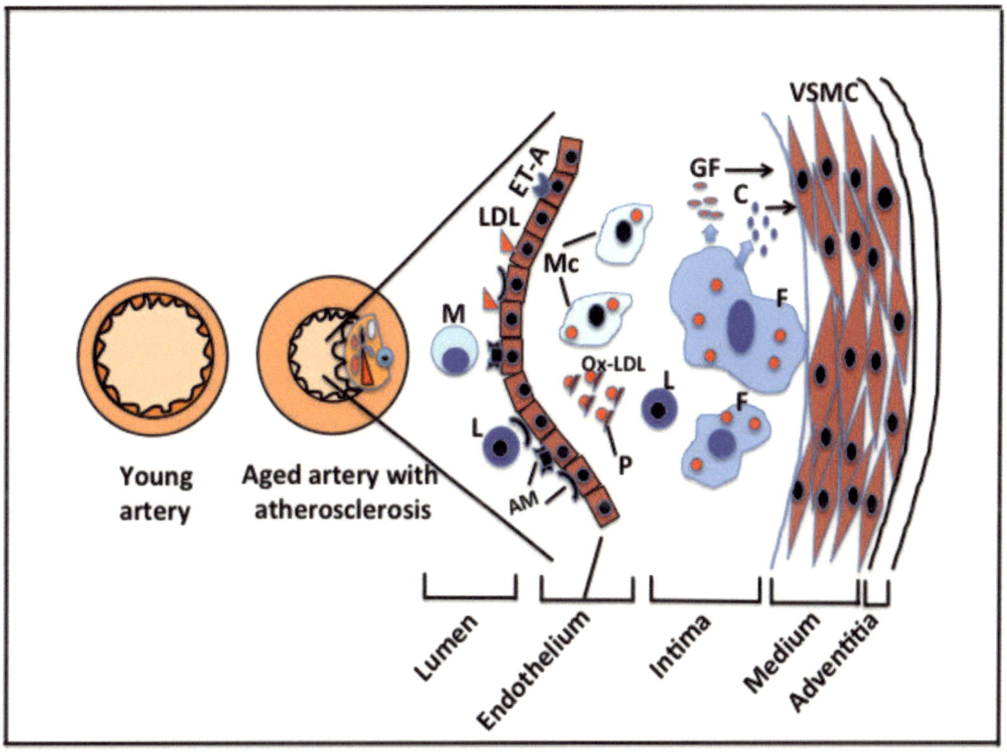

Figure 4. Atherosclerosis in the aged artery. Aged endothelial cells express various adhesion molecules (AM), which facilitate the binding as well as transportation of various inflammatory cells, including monocytes (M) and lymphocytes (L) into the intima. Oxidized low density lipoproteins (OxLDL) play a major role in the formation of foam cells (F). The foam cells secrete several growth factors (GF) and cytokines (C) that lead to increased proliferation of vascular smooth muscle cells (VSMCs). Increased expression of endothelin-1 facilitates atherosclerosis through ET-A receptor activation. The lymphocytes also play a critical role in causing inflammation in the endothelium. Altogether, these changes facilitate the plaque formation in the blood vessels of aged populations.

7.2. Diabetic retinopathy, a vascular disease of the eye

Diabetes affects approximately 200 million people around the world and almost 20 million in the United States. Diabetic retinopathy (DR) is a microvascular disease of the eye and most commonly seen in elderly population [72]. Type I as well as Type II diabetes lead to the development of DR. Importantly, microvessels of the eye are mostly affected by hyperglycemia. Several changes in the blood vessels have been observed including loss of pericytes, thickening of the basement membrane and increased permeability of blood vessels in DR. Furthermore, as DR progresses from non-proliferative DR to proliferative DR, the new blood vessels start to grow (neovascularization) to compensate for the affected blood vessels. Although the molecular mechanisms by which diabetes affects blood vessels of the eye remain not completely understood, it is evident from several studies that hyperglycemia directly plays a major role in causing DR. The highly elevated blood glucose activates aldose reductase pathway in certain tissues, which converts the sugars into alcohols, mainly sorbitol. The increased formation of sorbitol further affects the intramural pericytes present in the blood vessels of the retina to cause loss of function of pericytes [73]. As pericytes inhibit the endothelial cell function in occular blood vessels, loss of pericytes function leads to the formation of microaneurysms and ultimately lead to neovascularization. This pathological condition is mostly observed at the borders of retina and occurs along the vascular arcades as well as at the optic nerve head. The newly formed blood vessels do not directly affect the retina, however, the blood vessels are susceptible to vitreous traction and lead to hemorrhage into the vitreous cavity or preretinal space. If not treated, this condition may ultimately lead to vision loss. Many studies were attempted to understand the underlying molecular mechanisms by which neovascularization occurs in DR. Like in other pathological conditions described above, it is in part due to aging-associated defects in angiogenesis. Specifically, increased shear stress causes enhanced permeability of the blood vessels. On one hand, the blood vessels constantly remodel to adapt such changes induced by shear stress. On the other hand, the increased shear stress also causes activation, proliferation and migration of endothelial cells that ultimately cause neovascularization [74]. Furthermore, shear stress also known to cause vasodilatory effects by inhibiting endothelin1, a potent vasoconstrictor and increasing the levels of eNOS and prostaglandins which are potent vasodilators. Increased shear stress also increases matrix production by the endothelial cells, which causes basement thickening. Increased secretion of tissue-type plasminogen activator causes thrombosis and affects microcirculation [75]. Once blood vessels are obscured, the hypoxia generated inside will cause increased dilation of nearby vessels and leads to increased production of growth factors that further promote increased neovascularization.

Among the various growth factors, VEGF-A seems to be potentially involved in promoting angiogenesis in DR. In fact, Miller et al. demonstrated that increased VEGF-A levels correlate with enhanced angiogenesis in ocular tissue [76]. Moreover, high affinity receptors for VEGF-A have also been identified in endothelial cells as well as the pericytes of blood vessels located in the eye. This clearly suggests that VEGF-A-induced signaling pathway might play a potential role in promoting angiogenesis in DR. Furthermore, as angiogenesis is precisely regulated both by pro-angiogenic and anti-angiogenic factors, Funatsu et al. conducted studies to evaluate whether the balance between these two types of molecules is critical in causing angiogenesis in DR [77]. They simultaneously measured pro-angiogenic (VEGF-A) as well as anti-angiogenic molecules (endostatin and PF4) in the vitreous and in the plasma samples to correlate with DR. Interestingly, these studies revealed that vitreous VEGF-A and endostatin levels clearly correlate with the severity of DR, however, no correlation was found between DR and plasma levels of VEGF-A and endostatin [77]. Therefore, this study suggested that loss of balance between pro- and anti-angiogenic molecules might be responsible for the neovascularization observed in DR.

Several drugs were investigated to inhibit neovascularization associated with DR. For example, Ruboxistaurin, a protein kinase C inhibitor tested for efficacy. This is based upon the effects of hyperglycemia on diacylglycerol, which is known to be elevated in DR. Diacylglycerol is a potent activator of protein kinase C, and in turn protein kinase C increases VEGF-A secretion. The protein kinase C inhibitors are known to have some beneficial effects on DR. Furthermore, as VEGF-A levels are increased in DR, anti-VEGF-A compounds were also developed to specifically inhibit neovascularization associated with DR [78].

8. Conclusion

Aging is one of the major risk factors for the development of various vascular diseases such as cardiovascular disease, peripheral vascular disease and vascular diseases of the eye. Although exact molecular mechanisms are not clearly known, several molecules are known to be altered in aged endothelial cells. Importantly, reduced expression of eNOS and decreased production of NO, a potent vasodilator, have been observed. Furthermore, decreased expression of VEGF and VEGF receptors, and conversely, increased expression of TSP2, a potent angiogenesis inhibitor, have been observed in aged endothelial cells as well. The imbalance between the pro-angiogenic and the anti-angiogenic molecules seems to be responsible for the decreased angiogenesis observed in aged endothelial cells. Importantly, it has been also demonstrated that aging-induced oxidative stress is one of the major contributing factors for the loss of endothelial cell function in advanced age. In this regard, novel antioxidants may prevent aging-induced oxidative stress and thereby improve endothelial cell function in aged cells. As most of the pro-angiogenic and the anti-angiogenic molecules are unstable, recent studies have also established a potential role of UPS in regulating endothelial cell function. However, further thorough investigations are required to pinpoint the precise role of UPS in regulating the aging-associated decline of angiogenesis in the endothelial cells. To this end, it is critical to identify the age-associated molecular signature changes in different cells present in the endothelium such as endothelial cells, smooth muscle cells and pericytes in order to understand how these changes ultimately lead to the loss of endothelial function. This critical information will not only help to identify the crucial signaling pathways through which aging process affects the angiogenesis, but also will aid to develop novel therapies to combat various vascular diseases associated with aging.

Acknowledgements

This work is supported by the grants from National Institutes of Health to Wenyi Wei (GM089763; GM094777). Shavali Shaik and Zhiwei Wang are recipients of Ruth L. Kirschstein National Research Service Award (NRSA) fellowship. Hiroyuki Inuzuka is recipient of K01 award from National Institute on Aging, NIH (AG041218).

Author details

Shavali Shaik, Zhiwei Wang, Hiroyuki Inuzuka, Pengda Liu and Wenyi Wei*

Department of Pathology, Beth Israel Deaconess Medical Center, Harvard Medical School, Boston, MA, USA

Authors Shaik Shavali and Wang Zhiwei contributed equally to this work.

References

[1] Martin GM. The biology of aging: 1985-2010 and beyond. FASEB J 2011; 25 3756-3762.

[2] Wiener JM, Tilly J. Population ageing in the United States of America: implications for public programmes. Int J Epidemiol 2002; 31 776-781.

[3] North BJ, Sinclair DA. The intersection between aging and cardiovascular disease. Circ Res 2012; 110 1097.

[4] Lakatta EG. Age-associated cardiovascular changes in health: impact on cardiovascular disease in older persons. Heart Fail Rev 2002; 7 29-49.

[5] Kelly-Hayes M. Influence of age and health behaviors on stroke risk: lessons from longitudinal studies. J Am Geriatr Soc 2010; 58 Suppl 2 S325-328.

[6] Driver JA, Djousse L, Logroscino G, Gaziano JM, Kurth T. Incidence of cardiovascular disease and cancer in advanced age: prospective cohort study. BMJ 2008; 337 a2467.

[7] Sinclair DA, Guarente L. Unlocking the secrets of longevity genes. Sci Am 2006; 294 48-51, 54-47.

[8] Brown-Borg HM, Borg KE, Meliska CJ, Bartke. A Dwarf mice and the ageing process. Nature 1996; 384 33.

[9] Barzilai N, Huffman DM, Muzumdar RH, Bartke. A The critical role of metabolic pathways in aging. Diabetes 2012; 61 1315-1322.

[10] Wood JG, Rogina B, Lavu S, Howitz K, Helfand SL, et al. Sirtuin activators mimic caloric restriction and delay ageing in metazoans. Nature 2004; 430 686-689.

[11] Finkel T, Holbrook NJ. Oxidants, oxidative stress and the biology of ageing. Nature 2000; 408 239-247.

[12] Brandes RP, Fleming I, Busse R. Endothelial aging. Cardiovasc Res 2005; 66 286-294.

[13] Ungvari Z, Kaley G, de Cabo R, Sonntag WE, Csiszar A. Mechanisms of vascular aging: new perspectives. J Gerontol A Biol Sci Med Sci 2010; 65 1028-1041.

[14] Oxenham H, Sharpe N. Cardiovascular aging and heart failure. Eur J Heart Fail 2003; 5 427-434.

[15] Michiels C. Endothelial cell functions. J Cell Physiol 2003; 196 430-443.

[16] Neufeld G, Cohen T, Gengrinovitch S, Poltorak Z. Vascular endothelial growth factor (VEGF) and its receptors. FASEB J 1999; 13 9-22.

[17] Shalaby F, Rossant J, Yamaguchi TP, Gertsenstein M, Wu XF, et al. Failure of blood-island formation and vasculogenesis in Flk-1-deficient mice. Nature 1995; 376 62-66.

[18] Fleming I, Busse R. NO: the primary EDRF. J Mol Cell Cardiol 1999; 31 5-14.

[19] Kubes P, Suzuki M, Granger DN. Nitric oxide: an endogenous modulator of leukocyte adhesion. Proc Natl Acad Sci U S A 1991; 88 4651-4655.

[20] Mellion BT, Ignarro LJ, Ohlstein EH, Pontecorvo EG, Hyman AL, et al. Evidence for the inhibitory role of guanosine 3', 5'-monophosphate in ADP-induced human platelet aggregation in the presence of nitric oxide and related vasodilators. Blood 1981; 57 946-955.

[21] Garg UC, Hassid A. Nitric oxide-generating vasodilators and 8-bromo-cyclic guanosine monophosphate inhibit mitogenesis and proliferation of cultured rat vascular smooth muscle cells. J Clin Invest 1989; 83 1774-1777.

[22] Lyons D, Roy S, Patel M, Benjamin N, Swift CG. Impaired nitric oxide-mediated vasodilatation and total body nitric oxide production in healthy old age. Clin Sci (Lond) 1997; 93 519-525.

[23] Tanabe T, Maeda S, Miyauchi T, Iemitsu M, Takanashi M, et al. Exercise training improves ageing-induced decrease in eNOS expression of the aorta. Acta Physiol Scand 2003; 178 3-10.

[24] Yoon HJ, Cho SW, Ahn BW, Yang SY. Alterations in the activity and expression of endothelial NO synthase in aged human endothelial cells. Mech Ageing Dev 2010; 131 119-123.

[25] Hamilton CA, Brosnan MJ, McIntyre M, Graham D, Dominiczak AF. Superoxide excess in hypertension and aging: a common cause of endothelial dysfunction. Hypertension 2001; 37 529-534.

[26] Csiszar A, Ungvari Z, Edwards JG, Kaminski P, Wolin MS, et al. Aging-induced phenotypic changes and oxidative stress impair coronary arteriolar function. Circ Res 2002; 90 1159-1166.

[27] Davis ME, Cai H, Drummond GR, Harrison DG. Shear stress regulates endothelial nitric oxide synthase expression through c-Src by divergent signaling pathways. Circ Res 2001; 89 1073-1080.

[28] Kleinert H, Wallerath T, Euchenhofer C, Ihrig-Biedert I, Li H, et al. Estrogens increase transcription of the human endothelial NO synthase gene: analysis of the transcription factors involved. Hypertension 1998; 31 582-588.

[29] Bouloumie A, Schini-Kerth VB, Busse R. Vascular endothelial growth factor up-regulates nitric oxide synthase expression in endothelial cells. Cardiovasc Res 1999; 41 773-780.

[30] Yildiz O. Vascular smooth muscle and endothelial functions in aging. Ann N Y Acad Sci 2007; 1100 353-360.

[31] Pugh CW, Ratcliffe PJ. Regulation of angiogenesis by hypoxia: role of the HIF system. Nat Med 2003; 9 677-684.

[32] Rivard A, Fabre JE, Silver M, Chen D, Murohara T, et al. Age-dependent impairment of angiogenesis. Circulation 1999; 99 111-120.

[33] Swift ME, Kleinman HK, DiPietro LA. Impaired wound repair and delayed angiogenesis in aged mice. Lab Invest 1999; 79 1479-1487.

[34] Thomasona HA, Hardman MJ. Delayed wound healing in elderly people. Reviews in Clinical Gerontology 2009; 19 171.

[35] Qian HS, de Resende MM, Beausejour C, Huw LY, Liu P, et al. Age-dependent acceleration of ischemic injury in endothelial nitric oxide synthase-deficient mice: potential role of impaired VEGF receptor 2 expression. J Cardiovasc Pharmacol 2006; 47 587-593.

[36] Agah A, Kyriakides TR, Letrondo N, Bjorkblom B, Bornstein P. Thrombospondin 2 levels are increased in aged mice: consequences for cutaneous wound healing and angiogenesis. Matrix Biol 2004; 22 539-547.

[37] Vasa M, Breitschopf K, Zeiher AM, Dimmeler S. Nitric oxide activates telomerase and delays endothelial cell senescence. Circ Res 2000; 87 540-542.

[38] Yang J, Chang E, Cherry AM, Bangs CD, Oei Y, et al. Human endothelial cell life extension by telomerase expression. J Biol Chem 1999; 274 26141-26148.

[39] Matsushita H, Chang E, Glassford AJ, Cooke JP, Chiu CP, et al. eNOS activity is reduced in senescent human endothelial cells: Preservation by hTERT immortalization. Circ Res 2001; 89 793-798.

[40] Murasawa S, Llevadot J, Silver M, Isner JM, Losordo DW, et al. Constitutive human telomerase reverse transcriptase expression enhances regenerative properties of endothelial progenitor cells. Circulation 2002; 106 1133-1139.

[41] Watanabe Y, Lee SW, Detmar M, Ajioka I, Dvorak HF .Vascular permeability factor/ vascular endothelial growth factor (VPF/VEGF) delays and induces escape from senescence in human dermal microvascular endothelial cells. Oncogene 1997; 14 2025-2032.

[42] Donato AJ, Eskurza I, Silver AE, Levy AS, Pierce GL, et al. Direct evidence of endothelial oxidative stress with aging in humans: relation to impaired endothelium-dependent dilation and upregulation of nuclear factor-kappaB. Circ Res 2007; 100 1659-1666.

[43] Francia P, delli Gatti C, Bachschmid M, Martin-Padura I, Savoia C, et al. Deletion of p66shc gene protects against age-related endothelial dysfunction. Circulation 2004; 110 2889-2895.

[44] van der Loo B, Labugger R, Skepper JN, Bachschmid M, Kilo J, et al. Enhanced peroxynitrite formation is associated with vascular aging. J Exp Med 2000; 192 1731-1744.

[45] Furumoto K, Inoue E, Nagao N, Hiyama E, Miwa N. Age-dependent telomere shortening is slowed down by enrichment of intracellular vitamin C via suppression of oxidative stress. Life Sci 1998; 63 935-948.

[46] Haendeler J, Hoffmann J, Diehl JF, Vasa M, Spyridopoulos I, et al. Antioxidants inhibit nuclear export of telomerase reverse transcriptase and delay replicative senescence of endothelial cells. Circ Res 2004; 94 768-775.

[47] Zhou S, Chen HZ, Wan YZ, Zhang QJ, Wei YS, et al. Repression of P66Shc expression by SIRT1 contributes to the prevention of hyperglycemia-induced endothelial dysfunction. Circ Res 2011; 109 639-648.

[48] Yusuf S, Dagenais G, Pogue J, Bosch J, Sleight P. Vitamin E supplementation and cardiovascular events in high-risk patients. The Heart Outcomes Prevention Evaluation Study Investigators. N Engl J Med 2000; 342 154-160.

[49] Sesso HD, Buring JE, Christen WG, Kurth T, Belanger C, et al. Vitamins E and C in the prevention of cardiovascular disease in men: the Physicians' Health Study II randomized controlled trial. JAMA 2008; 300 2123-2133.

[50] Hershko A, Ciechanover A. The ubiquitin system. Annu Rev Biochem 1998; 67 425-479.

[51] Shaik S, Liu P, Fukushima H, Wang Z, Wei W. Protein degradation in cell cycle. In: eLS John Wiley & Sons Ltd, Chichester (UK) 2012.

[52] Jiang J, Cyr D, Babbitt RW, Sessa WC, Patterson C. Chaperone-dependent regulation of endothelial nitric-oxide synthase intracellular trafficking by the co-chaperone/ubiquitin ligase CHIP. J Biol Chem 2003; 278 49332-49341.

[53] Musial A, Eissa NT. Inducible nitric-oxide synthase is regulated by the proteasome degradation pathway. J Biol Chem 2001; 276 24268-24273.

[54] Ohh M, Park CW, Ivan M, Hoffman MA, Kim TY, et al. Ubiquitination of hypoxia-inducible factor requires direct binding to the beta-domain of the von Hippel-Lindau protein. Nat Cell Biol 2000; 2 423-427.

[55] Stangl V, Lorenz M, Meiners S, Ludwig A, Bartsch C, et al. Long-term up-regulation of eNOS and improvement of endothelial function by inhibition of the ubiquitin-proteasome pathway. FASEB J 2004; 18 272-279.

[56] Tsunematsu R, Nakayama K, Oike Y, Nishiyama M, Ishida N, et al. Mouse Fbw7/Sel-10/Cdc4 is required for notch degradation during vascular development. J Biol Chem 2004; 279 9417-9423.

[57] Tetzlaff MT, Yu W, Li M, Zhang P, Finegold M, et al. Defective cardiovascular development and elevated cyclin E and Notch proteins in mice lacking the Fbw7 F-box protein. Proc Natl Acad Sci U S A 2004; 101 3338-3345.

[58] Shaik S, Nucera C, Inuzuka H, Gao D, Garnaas M, et al. SCFbeta-TRCP suppresses angiogenesis and thyroid cancer cell migration by promoting ubiquitination and destruction of VEGF receptor 2. J Exp Med 2012; 209 1289-1307.

[59] Fleg JL, Aronow WS, Frishman WH. Cardiovascular drug therapy in the elderly: benefits and challenges. Nat Rev Cardiol 2011; 8 13-28.

[60] Goettsch W, Lattmann T, Amann K, Szibor M, Morawietz H, et al. Increased expression of endothelin-1 and inducible nitric oxide synthase isoform II in aging arteries in vivo: implications for atherosclerosis. Biochem Biophys Res Commun 2001; 280 908-913.

[61] d'Uscio LV, Barton M, Shaw S, Luscher TF. Endothelin in atherosclerosis: importance of risk factors and therapeutic implications. J Cardiovasc Pharmacol 2000; 35 S55-59.

[62] Amiri F, Virdis A, Neves MF, Iglarz M, Seidah NG, et al. Endothelium-restricted overexpression of human endothelin-1 causes vascular remodeling and endothelial dysfunction. Circulation 2004; 110 2233-2240.

[63] Barton M, Haudenschild CC, d'Uscio LV, Shaw S, Munter K, et al. Endothelin ETA receptor blockade restores NO-mediated endothelial function and inhibits atherosclerosis in apolipoprotein E-deficient mice. Proc Natl Acad Sci U S A 1998; 95 14367-14372.

[64] Wedgwood S, Black SM. Endothelin-1 decreases endothelial NOS expression and activity through ETA receptor-mediated generation of hydrogen peroxide. Am J Physiol Lung Cell Mol Physiol 2005; 288 L480-487.

[65] Morisaki N, Saito I, Tamura K, Tashiro J, Masuda M, et al. New indices of ischemic heart disease and aging: studies on the serum levels of soluble intercellular adhesion molecule-1 (ICAM-1) and soluble vascular cell adhesion molecule-1 (VCAM-1) in patients with hypercholesterolemia and ischemic heart disease. Atherosclerosis 1997; 131 43-48.

[66] Hansson GK. Inflammation, atherosclerosis, and coronary artery disease. N Engl J Med 2005; 352 1685-1695.

[67] del Rincon ID, Williams K, Stern MP, Freeman GL, Escalante. A High incidence of cardiovascular events in a rheumatoid arthritis cohort not explained by traditional cardiac risk factors. Arthritis Rheum 2001; 44 2737-2745.

[68] Del Rincon I, Williams K, Stern MP, Freeman GL, O'Leary DH, et al. Association between carotid atherosclerosis and markers of inflammation in rheumatoid arthritis patients and healthy subjects. Arthritis Rheum 2003; 48 1833-1840.

[69] Roman MJ, Shanker BA, Davis A, Lockshin MD, Sammaritano L, et al. Prevalence and correlates of accelerated atherosclerosis in systemic lupus erythematosus. N Engl J Med 2003; 349 2399-2406.

[70] Hallenbeck JM, Hansson GK, Becker KJ. Immunology of ischemic vascular disease: plaque to attack. Trends Immunol 2005; 26 550-556.

[71] Vogt MT, Wolfson SK, Kuller LH. Lower extremity arterial disease and the aging process: a review. J Clin Epidemiol 1992; 45 529-542.

[72] Paulus YM, Gariano RF. Diabetic retinopathy: a growing concern in an aging population. Geriatrics 2009; 64 16-20.

[73] Orlidge A, D'Amore PA. Inhibition of capillary endothelial cell growth by pericytes and smooth muscle cells. J Cell Biol 1987; 105 1455-1462.

[74] Ando J, Nomura H, Kamiya A. The effect of fluid shear stress on the migration and proliferation of cultured endothelial cells. Microvasc Res 1987; 33 62-70.

[75] Iba T, Shin T, Sonoda T, Rosales O, Sumpio BE. Stimulation of endothelial secretion of tissue-type plasminogen activator by repetitive stretch. J Surg Res 1991; 50 457-460.

[76] Miller JW, Adamis AP, Shima DT, D'Amore PA, Moulton RS, et al. Vascular endothelial growth factor/vascular permeability factor is temporally and spatially correlated with ocular angiogenesis in a primate model. Am J Pathol 1994; 145 574-584.

[77] Funatsu H, Yamashita H, Noma H, Mochizuki H, Mimura T, et al. Outcome of vitreous surgery and the balance between vascular endothelial growth factor and endostatin. Invest Ophthalmol Vis Sci 2003; 44 1042-1047.

[78] Bhavsar AR. Diabetic retinopathy: the latest in current management. Retina 2006; 26 S71-79.

Section 2

Cellular Senescence

Chapter 2

Molecular Mechanisms of Cellular Senescence

Therese Becker and Sebastian Haferkamp

Additional information is available at the end of the chapter

http://dx.doi.org/10.5772/54120

1. Introduction

Normal mammalian cells in culture have a limited life span and will eventually maintain a growth arrested state, referred to as replicative senescence. Usually induced by telomere shortening this form of arrest is irreversible in the sense that cells cannot be triggered to re-enter proliferation by physiological mitotic stimuli like growth factors. Senescence may also occur prematurely in response to various stress stimuli such as oxidative stress, DNA damage or active oncogenes. Thereby premature senescence acts as an important tumor suppressive mechanism and not surprisingly there is emerging evidence that senescence is indeed not only a result of tissue culture but markers of senescence have been identified in vivo in human and animal tissue.

The function of the retinoblastoma protein (pRb) is central to the onset of senescence. pRb, in its active hypophosphorylated form, is a potent repressor of genes that function during DNA replication and thereby pRb causes cell cycle arrest. The cell cycle inhibitors $p16^{INK4a}$ and $p21^{Waf1}$ and their homologues work in concert with pRb by inhibiting cyclin dependent kinases (CDKs) from phosphorylating pRb and thus maintaining in its active growth inhibitory state.

Additionally to the transient role in growth inhibition active, hypophosphorylated pRb coordinates major changes in direct and epigenetic gene regulation leading to changes in chromatin structure, which are crucial to the onset and maintenance of senescence.

This chapter provides an insight in these molecular mechanisms of cellular senescence.

2. Senescence features and biomarkers

Senescent cells display several characteristic morphological and biochemical features. The detection of these markers has been used to identify senescent cells in vitro an in vivo. The typical senescence phenotype consist of enlarged cell with multiple or enlarged nuclei, prominent Golgi apparatus and sometimes a vacuolated cytoplasm (Figure1). Recently a novel method to measure protein levels with fluorescence microscopy confirmed that indeed senescent cells accumulate increased levels of protein in the cytoplasm and nucleus [1]. In addition to the detection of characteristic morphological changes the most common method used to identify senescent cells is measurement of the lysosomal beta-galactosidase activity with a simple biochemical assay [2]. Due to an expansion of the lysosomes senescent cells show an increased activity of this enzyme, which is therefore often referred to as senescence-associated beta-galactosidase (SA-beta-gal), [3, 4]. However, it should be noted, that an increased beta-gal activity is an unreliable marker of senescence since it is also detectable in vitro after prolonged cell culture, serum withdrawal, TGF-beta, heparin or TPA treatment [3, 5-8]. The tumour suppressors $p16^{INK4a}$ and $p21^{Waf1}$ are mediators of cell cycle arrest and senescence and therefore often used as biomarkers. Since neither $p16^{INK4a}$ nor $p21^{Waf1}$ is strictly required for the induction or maintenance of the senescence program their predictive value is limited if used individually. A specific feature of senescent cells are condensed heterochromatic regions, known as senescence-associated heterochromatic foci (SAHF). These heterochromatin spots are enriched with i) histone H3-methylated at lysine 9 (H3K9meth), its binding partner ii) heterochromatin protein-1γ (HP- 1γ) and iii) the non-histone chromatin protein, HMGA2, which all have been used as markers of SAHF [9, 10].

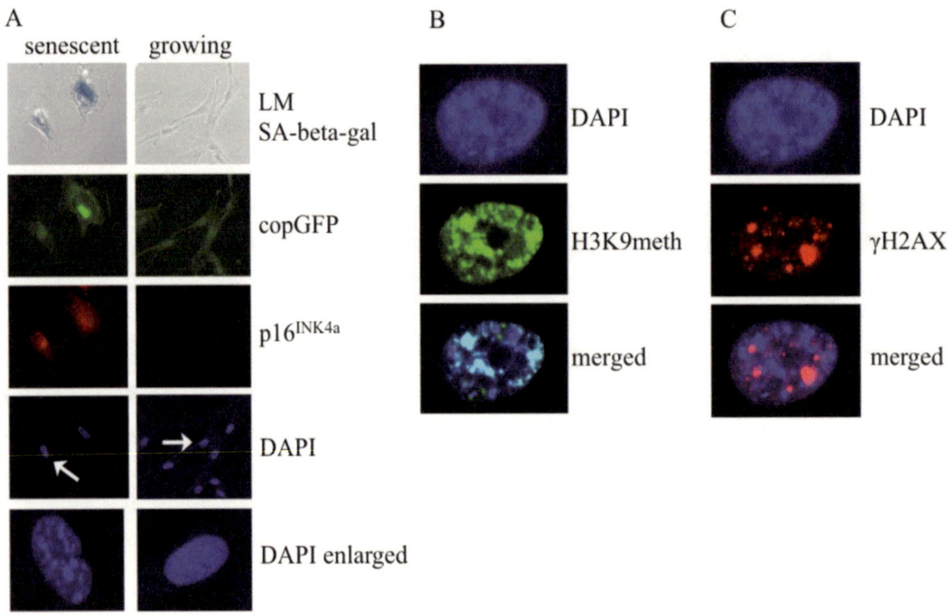

Figure 1. Senescence characteristics

A) The typical senescence phenotype consist of enlarged cell with multiple or enlarged nuclei, and an increased SA-beta-gal activity is visible after N-RAS^{Q61K} induced senescence. Human diploid fibroblasts (HDF) were transduced with lentiviruses expressing N-RAS^{Q61K} or copGFP control. The efficiency of transduction was controlled with the co-expression of copGFP and was consistently above 90%. p16^{Ink4a} expression, chromatin condensation (DAPI), and the appearance of increased SA-ß-Gal activity were analyzed and quantified 15 days after infection. Cells enlarged to show DAPI-stained chromatin foci are indicated with arrows. B, C) HDF induced to senesce with oncogenic N-RAS^{Q61K} were stained with DAPI and an antibody to H3K9meth or γH2AX to highlight senescence-associated heterochromatin foci or DNA damage foci respectively. H2AX is a member of the histone H2A family that gets instantly phosphorylated after DNA damage and forms foci at DNA break sites.

3. pRb in cell cycle regulation

The retinoblastoma protein (pRb) is often referred to as the "master brake" of the cell cycle because its main function is to inhibit E2F transcription factors from inducing a range of genes essential for DNA replication and thus proliferation [11]. Consequently active pRb causes cell cycle arrest. In contrast during proliferation when cells are promoted towards cell division, pRb is sequentially phosphorylated by a series of cyclin dependent kinases (CDKs) and this results in pRb inactivation and consequently derepression of proliferation genes.

Initiation of cell proliferation is normally triggered by growth factors. These external molecules function as ligands to a number of growth factor receptors expressed on the cell surface and thus activate signalling cascades, most prominently the mitogen activated protein kinase (MAPK) pathway, and ultimately lead to the expression of a number of genes including cyclin D [12]. CDK4 and 6 initiate phosphorylation of pRb in the presence of cyclin D and this leads to de-repression of early cell cycle genes including cyclin E and thus the entry into the cell cycle. Subsequently, CDK2 and CDK1, in co-operation with cyclins E, A and B, continue to stepwise further phosphorylate and inactivate pRb, which leads to cell cycle progression and finally cell division. As the "master brake" of the cell cycle pRb is an important tumor suppressor and alterations of its pathway have been associated with the childhood cancer retinoblastoma and are known to occur in over 90% of cancers [13]. There are two important types of cell cycle inhibitors represented most prominently by p16^{INK4a} and p21^{Waf1}. p16^{INK4a} is at the forefront of cell cycle inhibition as it binds specifically to the cyclin D dependent kinases CDK4 and CDK6 and displaces cyclin D and thereby it prevents the entry into the cell cycle and arrests cells in G1 phase (Figure 2). p21^{Waf1} is more promiscuous and is able to inhibit all CDK molecules at any stage during the cell cycle. p21^{Waf1} molecules do not necessarily displace cyclin partners from their CDK target and importantly it may require several p21^{Waf1} molecules to effectively inhibit CDKs [14]. In normal cells p16^{INK4a} and p21^{Waf1} are able to work hand in hand, the accumulation of p16^{INK4a} and binding to CDK4 and 6 frees p21^{Waf1} molecules from these kinases to bind and inhibit CDK2 and 1 more efficiently [15]. These basic cell cycle regulatory functions of pRb, p16^{INK4a} and p21^{Waf1} are essential to initiate and maintain senescence and it is not surprising that all three molecules are considered important tumor suppressors.

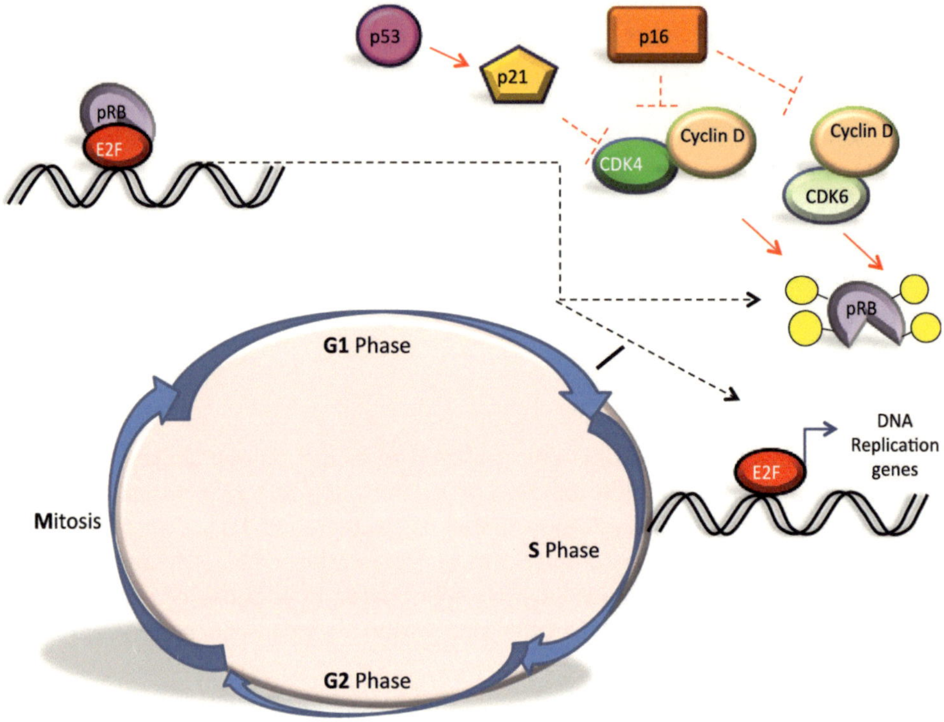

Figure 2. The Cell Cycle

This simplified model, focusing on early cell cycle entry, illustrates that hypophosphorylated, active pRb represses E2F-mediated transcription. The action of CDKs, exemplified by the cyclin D dependent CDK4 and 6, phosphorylate pRb and thus release E2F to activate transcription of early DNA replication genes. $p16^{INK4a}$ and $p21^{Waf1}$, the latter usually activated by p53, inhibit CDKs and retain pRb in its active cell cycle inhibitory state.

4. The role of the tumor suppressor p16INK4a in senescence

With regard to senescence, it is long known that $p16^{INK4a}$ levels accumulate and cause growth arrest and senescence when cells approach their replicative life span [16-23]. Moreover, in long term tissue culture studies cells that were able to overcome senescence commonly had lost $p16^{INK4a}$ and p53 expression [24]. Increased $p16^{INK4a}$ expression is also linked to oncogene induced and other forms of premature senescence [25-33].

Interestingly, despite this clear correlation of $p16^{INK4a}$ up-regulation with senescence there is some evidence from $p16^{INK4a}$ is not strictly required for senescence to occur. Evidence form mouse models show that mouse embryonic fibroblasts (MEFs) of p16-null mice undergo a comparable number of cell divisions as wild type MEFs before entering senescence [34] [35], while in primary melanocytes, which were lentivirally transduced to express oncogenic

HRAS or NRAS, silencing of $p16^{INK4a}$ did not abolish most senescent features. Interestingly however, the formation of SAHF did only occur in the presence of $p16^{INK4a}$ [29, 36, 37]. These findings show two important points: first there are other redundant mechanisms able to compensate for $p16^{INK4a}$ loss and rescue senescence and second the $p16^{INK4a}$-pRb pathway has a specific role in SAHF formation and, importantly, these heterochromatin foci have been suggested to abolish expression of proliferation associated genes and secure senescent features so senescence becomes irreversible [9] (see section 7 for more detail). This idea is supported by a report that senescence was only reversible, via p53 inactivation, in fibroblasts and mammary epithelial cells with low but not with high $p16^{INK4a}$ expression [38]. It is noteworthy that the importance of SAHF in securing senescence has been challenged recently and SAHF are thought dispensable for senescence by some investigators and/or only associated with oncogene-induced senescence [39, 40]. The fact that SAHF formation only occurs in the presence of increased $p16^{INK4a}$ levels remains undebated and it is therefore tempting to speculate a direct $p16^{INK4a}$ role in the formation of these structures.

Even though cells may be able to compensate for $p16^{INK4a}$ loss and still undergo a growth arrest characterised by most if not all senescent features, the importance of the tumor suppressor $p16^{INK4a}$ in senescence is clear as p16-null tumor cells can be driven into senescence by the sole re-expression of $p16^{INK4a}$: Induced $p16^{INK4a}$ expression in glioma cells caused a typical senescent phenotype [41], reversing promoter hypermethylation allowed for the re-expression of endogenous $p16^{INK4a}$ in oral squamous cell carcinoma cells leading to senescence [42], inducible $p16^{INK4a}$ expression in osteosarcoma cells induced senescence after 3-6 days, potentially irreversible after 6 days [43] and inducible $p16^{INK4a}$ in human melanoma cells caused a senescent phenotype after 3-5 days in the absence of p53 [44, 45]. Moreover, even in normal early passage human fibroblasts the ectopic introduction of $p16^{INK4a}$ or functional peptides thereof initiated cell cycle arrest and senescent features [46, 47]. In line with this, melanoma associated germline mutations of $p16^{INK4a}$ are impaired in inducing a cellular senescence program in melanoma cells and this disability to promote senescence may contribute to the melanoma-risk of $p16^{INK4a}$ linked melanoma-prone families [45].

5. Timing of Senescence by repression and activation of $p16^{INK4a}$

5.1. $p16^{INK4a}$ repression

In fact, the ability to induce senescence in response to accumulated or sudden genomic stress is probably the most important tumor suppressive function of $p16^{INK4a}$. In line with this consideration it is not surprising that $p16^{INK4a}$ expression is tightly repressed at the chromatin and transcriptional level in "young" proliferating cells and in cells with extensive renewal capacities, such as stem cells. The polycomb protein Bmi1, which is also known as "stem cell factor" is facilitating repression of the INK4a locus at the chromatin level [48, 49]. Intriguingly, in a functional feedback loop, in human fibroblasts the Bmi1-mediated repression of $p16^{INK4a}$ requires active pRb and also H3K27 (histone 3/lysine 27] trimethylation facilitated by the histone methyltransferase EZH2 in concert with a second polycomb protein,

SUZ12 [50]. Crucially, Bmi1 chromatin binding can be inhibited by its phosphorylation through the MAPK and p38 signalling pathways [51]. Hence these pathways are able to directly oppose p16^{INK4a} repression and lead to its transcriptional activation via Ets and Sp-1 during oncogene-induced senescence.

In concert with Bmi-linked chromatin-remodelling events a number of transcription factors facilitate p16^{INK4a} repression during the proliferative life-time of cells. The perhaps most important transcriptional repressors of p16^{INK4a} are Id proteins, with the main representative Id1. Id proteins function by binding to E-box DNA sequences to repress the INK4a promoter and importantly by interfering with Ets transcriptional complex formation and thereby inhibiting the main INK4a transcriptional activator, Ets, in two ways [52, 53]. In line with this, high Id1 levels were associated with early stage melanoma whereas premalignant and interestingly also more advanced melanoma showed limited Id1 expression [54]. This suggests a role of the Id1/ p16^{INK4a} regulative connection during melanomagenesis and Id1 may be dispensable in later melanoma stages once p16^{INK4a} is either more tightly repressed by engaging repressive histone modifications or inactivated by other mechanisms. Id1 down-regulation on the other hand is usually associated with cell differentiation and senescence [55]. Consequently, ectopic expression of Id1 delayed senescence in melanocytes [56] and keratinocytes [57], while MEFs lacking Id1 prematurely senesced due to increased p16^{INK4a} levels [58, 59]. Another way to oppose Ets driven p16^{INK4a} transcription was identified, when Cdh1, an adaptor protein of the anaphase promoting complex, was shown to bind to and promote degradation of Ets2 and thereby increased the replicative life span of MEFs [60], while the Epstein-Barr virus protein LMP1 represses p16^{INK4a} by promoting the nuclear export of Ets2 [61, 62]

Interestingly, p16^{INK4a} may also be repressed by the oncogene β-catenin, which has been linked to melanoma. β-catenin binds the INK4a promoter at a conservative β-catenin/Lef/Tcf binding site and thereby directly represses its transcription. Consequently β-catenin silencing increased p16^{INK4a} levels in A375P human melanoma cells, while stabilization of β-catenin together with oncogenic N-RAS led to prevention of senescence and thus, immortalization [63]. Importantly, a role of β-catenin in melanocyte senescence is controversial as nuclear β-catenin was commonly found in benign melanocytic nevi [64-66] and these lesions were proposed to be senescent by some investigators [29, 67], this again is controversial, as benign nevi are not be distinguished from normal melanocytes or primary melanomas using a range of common senescence markers [68]. It would clearly be interesting to test whether nuclear β-catenin does overlap with the expression of p16^{INK4a} in benign nevi as the latter is mosaic and not found in all cells [29] and co-localisation or lack of it could help clarify this debate. Another repressor of p16^{INK4a} is the "T-box transcription factor" Tbx2, this transcription factor binds to corresponding T-box DNA sequence elements [69]. Tbx2 overexpression was identified in melanomas and associated with melanoma progression [70].

5.2. p16^{INK4a} expression

When cells reach their finite life span the pendulum at the INK4a promoter swings from repression to activation and the SWI/SNF chromatin remodeling complex, replaces Bmi1 repressors and relaxes chromatin structures around the INK4 promoter region, which is strictly dependent on the SWI/SNF subunits BRG1 and hSnf5, and the relaxed chromatin structure allows transcription factor access [71] (Figure 3a). Alterations of hSnf5 are associated with early childhood rhabdoid cancer and re-expression of hSnf5 in rhabdoid cancer cells leads to p16^{INK4a} accumulation, growth arrest and senescence [71, 72] and this requires functional p16^{INK4a} [73].

The best understood transcription factors driving p16^{INK4a} expression and thereby growth arrest and senescence are Ets1 and Ets2. They are effectors of MAPK signalling, often in response to oncogenic stress, such as activating N-RAS or B-RAF mutations, which induce an increase in p16^{INK4a} levels [25, 29, 37, 52]. In line with this, human fibroblasts with biallelic mutations in p16^{INK4a} did increase mutant p16^{INK4a} expression in response to RAS signaling or expression of ectopic Ets, but failed to arrest or undergo senescence [74]. Interestingly increased p16^{INK4a} expression has also been linked to loss of p53 and this appears to be correlated with increased Ets protein half-life [75]. Another member of the Ets transcription factor family, ESE-3, was independently identified as a down stream target of p38 signalling and caused senescence via p16^{INK4a} up-regulation [76]. p38 signalling has been linked to enhanced p16^{INK4a} expression before and this involved the downstream transcription factor Sp-1, which was proposed to be required for p16^{INK4a} up-regulation during senescence in human fibroblasts [77]. Sp-1 was reported to engage the p300 enhancer leading to further p16^{INK4a} upregulation [78] (Figure 3b).

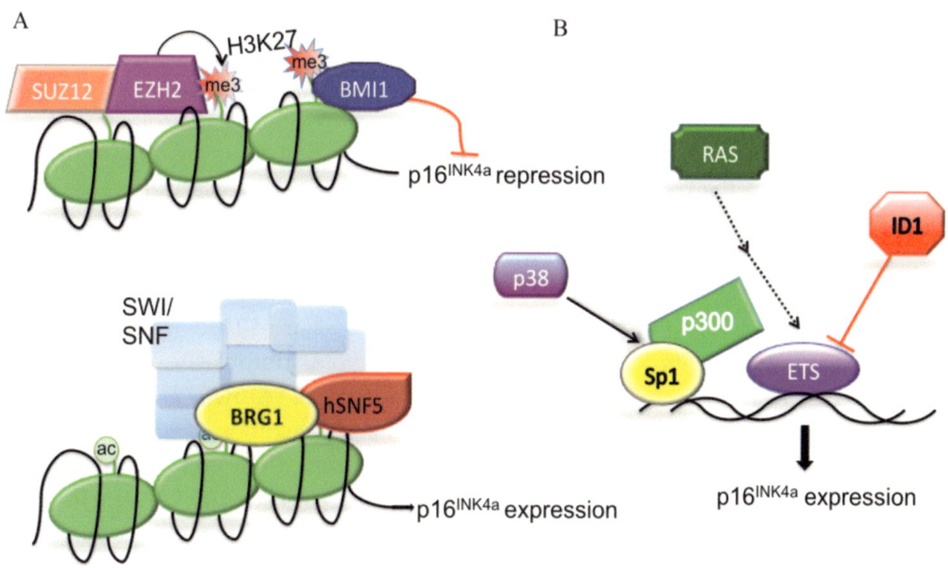

Figure 3. Schematic presentation of p16^{INK4a} regulation

(A) During the proliferative cellular life-time, EZH2 in cooperation with SUZ12 trimethylates H3K27 at the genomic INK4a locus and these histone modifications attract the polycomb repressor BMI1, which maintains the p16^{INK4a} promoter region inaccessible for transcriptional activation. Once cells reach their finite life span or during premature senescence the histone modifications at the INK4a locus change from repressive methylations to activating acetylations, which attract the SWI/SNF complex. The SWI/SNF subunits hSnf5 and BRG1 are instrumental in opening the chromatin structure and allowing access of the transcriptional machinery to the $p16^{INK4a}$ promoter. (B) Ets transcription factors are down stream targets of MAPK signalling, exemplified here by RAS, and bind to E-box $p16^{INK4}$ promoter motifs to activate gene expression. Id transcription factors can compete with Ets for DNA binding and oppose transcriptional expression. The levels of Id proteins decline with onset of senescence and Ets are able to promote $p16^{INK4a}$ expression.

6. The role of the p53/p21 pathway in senescence

The transcription factor and tumor suppressor p53 is often referred to as "guardian of the genome" and inactivating mutations in p53 are observed in about half of all human cancer cases. The p53 protein is a critical regulator of cell survival in response to cellular stress signals including DNA damage, oncogene activation, hypoxia and viral infection (reviewed in [79]. In the absence of stress stimuli p53 gets rapidly ubiquitinated by one of several E3 ligases including MDM2, MDM4, TOPORS, COP1, and ARF-BP1 and subsequently degraded in the proteasome [80, 81]. Stress signals, on the other hand, induce covalent modification usually by disrupting the interaction between p53 and the E3 ubiquitin ligases which prevents its degradation. Oncogenic stress, for example, activates the alternative reading frame product of the INK4a locus (p14ARF) that stabilizes p53 by binding and thereby inhibiting its negative regulator MDM2.

Several lines of evidence show convincingly that the p53 and its downstream effector $p21^{Waf1}$ play a crucial role in the regulation of cell cycle arrest and senescence. Overexpression of p53 [82] and $p21^{Waf1}$ [83-86] autonomously induced senescence in human cells and activation of p53 by either overexpression of p14ARF [87] or nutlin-3 treatment [88] induced senescence in a $p21^{Waf1}$ dependent manner in human diploid fibroblasts (HDF) and human glioblastoma cells respectively. Furthermore, inactivation of p53 or p19ARF (mouse homologue of human p14ARF) prevents senescence in mouse embryonic fibroblasts (MEF) [89-91] and human fibroblast lacking p21Waf1 can bypass the senescence growth arrest [83]. Further supporting evidence comes from studies that show that, inactivation of p53 using viral oncoproteins, anti-p53 antibodies or anti-sense oligonucleotides can extend the replicative lifespan or even reverse the senescence growth arrest in human cells [38, 92-94]. However, it should be noted that although inactivation of the p53 pathway can weaken or even reverse the senescence arrest in some cells, there is emerging evidence that it fails to do so in cells with an activated $p16^{INK4a}$/pRb pathway [38, 95-97]. Despite the clear evidence of p53's role in promoting senescence a study conducted by Demidenko and co-workers suggested that p53 can also act as an inhibitor of senescence [98]. Surprisingly, p53 was able to reverse a $p16^{INK4a}$ and $p21^{Waf1}$ driven senescence response in human fibroblasts. Although the underlying mechanisms are not fully understood, inhibition of the mTor (mammalian target of rapamycin) pathway seems to be involved in the repression of cellular senescence [98-101].

6.1. DNA damage and senescence

The human genome is constantly exposed to genotoxic stress such as ultraviolet light, reactive oxygen species (ROS) as well as chemical and biological mutagens. To ensure the integrity of the genome cells have evolved a sophisticated safety system that can implement a cell cycle arrest to allow the repair of the incurred damage. The initial step in the complicated DNA damage repair process is the detection of DNA damage. The Mre11/Rad50/NBS1 (*MRN*) complex function as a DNA damage sensor is localized in nuclear foci at the sites of double strand breaks (DSBs) [102-104]. Here, the complex tethers DNA ends, processes and repairs free strands via endonuclease and exonuclease activities [105-107]. The MRN complex is also involved in the recruitment and activation of ATM (ataxia-telangiectasia mutated) and ATR (ATM and Rad3-related) protein kinases, which in turn activate checkpoint-1/2 (CHK1/2) kinases leading to phosphorylation and thereby stabilization of a variety of target genes including p53 [108]. In the case of irreparable damage, the cell will be permanently retracted from the pool of dividing cells by the induction of apoptosis or senescence (Figure 4] [109, 110].

6.2. Drug induced senescence

Several sources of genotoxic stress including cisplatin, cyclophosphamide, doxorubicine, taxol, vincristine, cytarabine, etoposide, hydroxyurea, bromodeoxyuridine, adriamycin, bleomycin mitomycin D, interferon beta, radiation, ROS, H2O2 have been used to trigger senescence-like growth arrest in vitro and in vivo allowing a detailed analysis of the underlying signaling events [28, 111-122]. The crosslining agent cisplatin, for example, induced senescence in primary human fibroblasts and HCT116 colon carcinoma cells in a p53 and dose dependent manner [123, 124]). Interestingly, treatment of HCT116 cells with low cisplatin concentrations lead to DNA damage and senescence whereas high drug concentrations induced apoptosis via superoxide production. Furthermore, in human lung cancer cells induced p53 expression enhanced the cytotoxic effect of cisplatin whereas $p21^{waf1}$ overexpression surprisingly lead to increased drug resistance [82]. Similarly, cisplatin-resistant human non-small cell lung cancer (NSCLC) cells could be sensitized to drug-induced senescence by re-expressing $p16^{Ink4a}$ [118]. Duale and co-workers compared changes in the gene expression profiles of a cisplatin treated human colon carcinoma cells (HCT116) and cell lines derived from testicular germ cell tumors (TGCTs). The systematic approach combining the acquired gene expression data and other publicly available microarray data identified 1794 genes that were differentially expressed including 29 senescence-related genes such as IGFBP 7, interleukin 1 and MAPK8 [125]. These findings highlight the notion that cellular response to chemotherapeutic agents is generally depending on the cellular context as well as the type and level of the stress signal.

6.3. Oncogene-induced senescence and DNA damage

In contrast to chemotherapeutic agents that directly damage the DNA, activated oncogenes do the harm by forcing the cell in uncontrolled, constitute replication cycles which leads to DNA replication stress and subsequent DNA damage [126, 127]. During this process DNA replication forks stall making the DNA more susceptible to single or double strand breaks.

The subsequent activation of the DNA damage response (DDR) machinery delays cell-cycle progression by initiation of the ATM/ATR-CHK1/2 pathway and stable knockdown of any one of these DDR genes was sufficient to bypass RAS induced senescence in human fibroblasts. Specifically, in the absence of ATM, ATR, Chk1 or Chk2, human fibroblasts continued to proliferate despite Ras expression, and BrdU incorporation increased from approximately 5% in the control sample to 15% in cells deficient for a DNA damage protein. Interestingly, the inhibition of both the p16INK4a and DNA damage pathway enhanced the effect and enabled over 60% of the cells to replicate DNA [126]. In a similar study, Bartkova and co-workers showed that the suppression of ATM or p53 allowed the MRC5 and BJ human fibroblasts to bypass oncogene-induced senescence using overexpressed Mos (an activator of the MAPK pathway) or Cdc6 (a DNA replication licensing factor). However, in this report p16INK4a depletion alone did not weaken the senescence response [127].

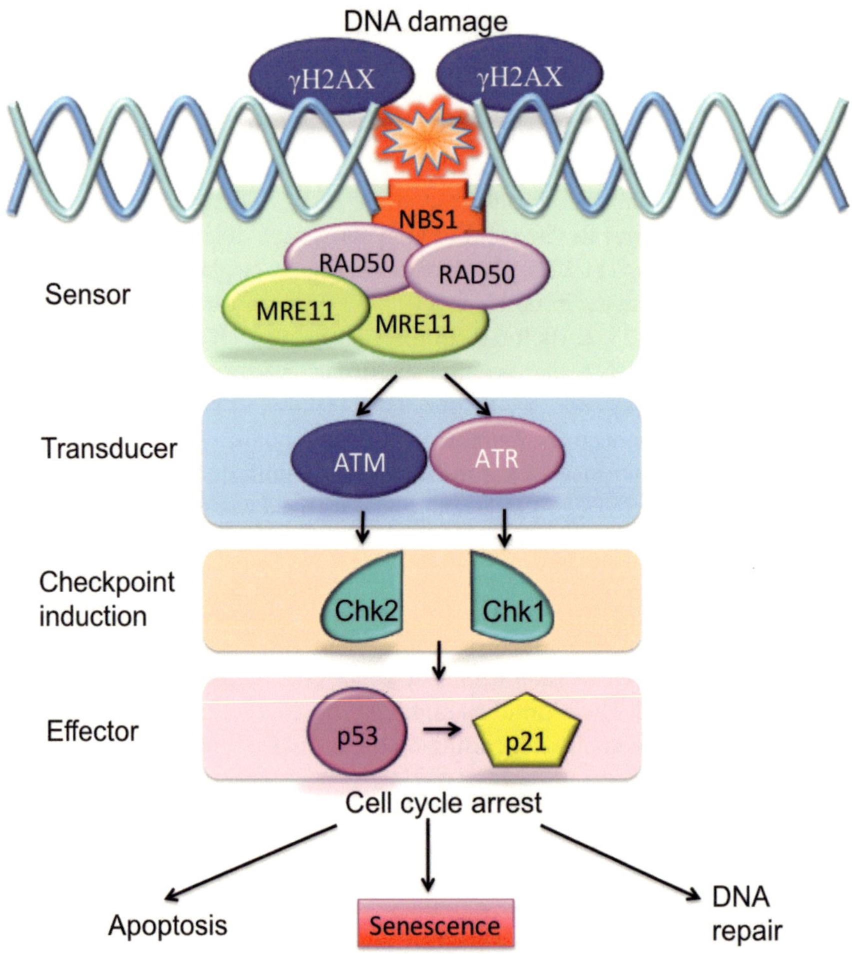

Figure 4. DNA damage pathway in senescence

To protect the integrity of their DNA, cells need to be able to sense DNA damage and activate response pathways that coordinate cell cycle progression and DNA repair. Ataxia telangiectasia mutated (ATM) and ATM-Rad3-related (ATR) kinases are important DNA damage checkpoints proteins that transduce signals from the DNA damage sensors to the effector proteins that control cell cycle progression, chromatin restructuring, and DNA repair. ATM and ATR activate other kinases such as Chkl (activated by ATR) and Chk2 (activated by ATM) that phosphorylate and activate the tumour suppressor protein p53. ATM and ATR can additionally enhance p53 activity by directing p53 phosphorylation on Ser15. Activated p53 can halt progression of the cell cycle in the G1 phase, allowing DNA repair to occur and preventing the transmission of damaged DNA to the daughter cells.

7. pRb in senescence: maintaining a secure proliferative arrest

In the previous sections we have reviewed the pivotal role of the cell cycle inhibitors $p16^{INK4a}$ and $p21^{Waf1}$ in keeping pRb in a hypophosphorylated, active state and explored the mechanisms of timing the expression of these tumor suppressors with the onset and maintenance of senescence. Here we explore the roles of active pRb in the senescence program, which go beyond the antiproliferative functions described in the cell cycle section 3.

There is longstanding evidence that pRb is required for an intact senescence program, for instance re-introduction of pRb into SAOS osteosarcoma cells that have lost its expression can cause senescence [128]. On the other hand inactivation of pRb with the viral oncoprotein E1A prevents senescence, while a mutant form of E1A that is impaired in pRb binding is unable to prevent senescence [9]. Interestingly, another mutant E1A, that is able to bind pRb but is unable to interact with the histone deacetylases p300 and p400 leads to less efficient development of senescence [9].

7.1. pRb and SAHFs

These data highlight that chromatin remodeling plays an important role in the cellular senescence program. Indeed, during senescence E2F responsive genomic promoter regions are stably repressed from transcription by the establishment of heterochromatin regions. As mentioned above (section 3) these regions are visible as microscopical "senescence associated heterochromatin foci" (SAHF) when cells are stained with certain DNA intercalating dyes such as DAPI. The term heterochromatin refers to a highly condensed protein-DNA structure, which is facilitated by modifications of the histone core molecules of chromatin and suppresses DNA access by the transcriptional machinery and thus gene expression of these regions is tightly suppressed (reviewed in [129]). The investigation of SAHF remains a progressing research field and is developing forward with improved microscopic imaging technology and the ability to isolate these complex structures and analyse them more precisely and we can expect to understand even more about their role and configuration in the future. To date we know that SAHF formation coincides with the recruitment of heterochromatin proteins by pRb when interacting with the histone deacetylase 1 (HDAC1] at E2F-responsive promoters [130]. A number of heterochromatin-associated histone modifications were characteristically found associated with SAHF. These include the reversion of histone 3/lysine 9 acetylation (H3K9Ac) and histone 3/lysine 4 trimethylation (H3K4me3) and significantly, since it is often used as a marker of senescence, the promotion of histone 3/lysine 9 trimethylation (H3K9me3) and H3K27me3. H3K9 trimethylation is a fundamental step during heterochromatin formation as it attracts HP1 proteins, which are pivotal for heterochromatin assembly [9]. It is important to highlight that senescence does not always lead to a net increase in overall H3K9me3, suggesting that SAHF formation is local and indeed targeted via pRb to E2F promoters [131]. H3K9me3 is thought to be very stable and is able to prevent histone acetylases (HATs) to catalyze histone acetylations. Histone acetylations are commonly associated with "euchromatin", which describes actively transcribed chromatin regions. Accordingly, SAHF formation is thought to "lock" chromatin regions that encode proliferation genes and thus contributes to the very secure silencing of E2F responsive proliferation genes, which is not reversible by physiological stimuli [9]. H3K9 trimethylation associated with SAHF formation is thought to be catalyzed by either the SUV39H1 methyltransferase, which together with HP1 interacts with pRb during E2F promoter silencing in senescence [132] or the RIZ1/PRDM2 H3K9 methyltransferase, which was also shown to co-operate in pRb gene repression and is inactivated in colon, breast and gastric carcinoma [133]. Furthermore, a search for H3K9me3 interacting proteins to identify proteins involved in the senescence program identified JMJD2C, which is a H3K9 specific demethylase. Thereby it is the direct antagonist of the SUV39H1 H3K9 methyltransferase and its over-expression is not surprisingly associated with several forms of cancer [134].

Lately there is a different view about the importance of SAHF emerging and SAHF formation, may according to a recent study only be of major relevance in the oncogene induced senescence process that crucially involves DDR and the corresponding ATR signalling, as knock-down of ATR prevents SAHF formation during RAS induced senescence. The same study also found that SAHF resembling structures containing H3K9me3 do independently occur in proliferating oncogene expressing cells, however the investigators data show that these structures are not associated with E2F target promoters, which remain active. The authors concluded that SAHF structures might not be an essential feature of senescence [40].

More recently a groundbreaking study by the Narita group has combined microscopic, electron microscopic and genomic data analysis to shed more light on SAHF formation and structure. Their significant findings are that H3K9me3 and H3K27me3 may in fact not directly be involved in SAHF. Although these markers are usually associated with SAHF, the overall methylation status of histone tail lysines does not change within the genomic DNA during senescence. Moreover, the investigators found that SAHF formation was linked to pre-senescent replication timing and specific histone modifications were characteristic for early-, mid- and late replications genes. Significantly though, when they prevented SAHF formation by silencing of either pRb or the high mobility group AT-hook 1 (HMGA-1), which they and others had previously linked to SAHF formation, there was no change to H3K9me3 in proliferating cells [135] and this may explain the above-mentioned data by Micco et al [40]. Moreover, Chandra et al. reversed H3K9 and H3K27 trimethylation by either overexpressing the H3K9me3 favoring histone demethlyase JMJD2D or by silencing SUZ12, a polycomb protein involved in H3K9 and K27 methylation. Importantly, even without these methylated histone markers RAS induction still led to senescence with the occurrence of DAPI dense SAHF structures. The investigators concluded that SAHF formation is mediated through spatial rearrangement of pre-existing H3K9me3 and H3K27me3 regions but that these histone marks are not a prerequisite for the SAHF formation process [135]. Clearly, further studies are needed to fully define the combined roles of histone modifications, heterochromatin and SAHF in senescence.

Consistent with gene silencing and decreased acetylation during senescence is the down-regulation of the histone acetylases p300/CBP, which was observed in melanocytes reaching in their finitive lifespan [136].

With regard to the role of chromatin remodelling in senescence, there is also evidence that ATP dependent chromatin remodeling complexes, such as SWI/SNF are required for senescence onset in roles other than the timely expression of p16INK4a as described in section 5.1.2: The introduction of the ATPase active component of the SWI/SNF complex, BRG1, into various cell lines induced senescent features. This is attributed to the BRG1 ability to interact with pRb and participate in E2F target promopter repression [137]. However development of senescence in response to BRG1 introduction was only convincing in cells that also lack the BRG1 homologue ATPase BRM [138]. Interestingly we found that BRG1 is able to interact with $p16^{INK4a}$, and since $p16^{INK4a}$ is required for SAHF formation it might directly be involved in this process in co-operation with BRG1. However, the absence of BRG1, by specific silencing, does neither prevent $p16^{INK4a}$ induced growth arrest nor senescence associated SAHF formation. It should be noted however, that the WMM1175 melanoma cells used in these experiments also express the BRG1 homologue BRM and therefore they still have functional SWI/SNF complexes even in the absence of BRG1. [139]. It still needs to be tested whether BRM also interacts with $p16^{INK4a}$ and whether the BRM-$p16^{INK4a}$ complex is involved in SAHF formation. This idea is in line with a suggested role for BRM in melanocyte senescence as it was demonstrated that BRM was recruited and required, albeit transiently, by the pRb-HDAC1 complex during the initiation of SAHF [140].

Importantly, although the p53-p21 pathway was demonstrated to be capable of inducing a number of senescent features and does so in response to DNA damage, telomere dysfunction and oncogene induced senescence [38, 97], E2F promoter silencing via SAHF formation requires an intact p16-pRb pathway [9, 141]. As expected, SAHF formation is prevented by cancer associated $p16^{INK4a}$ mutations [45]. Since p21Waf1 is capable of inhibiting all CDKs it remains unclear why it appears less effective in promoting a secure senescence program in involving heterochromatin formation (Figure5).

The current view is that pRb binds HDAC1 and attracts H3K9 and H3K27 methylating complexes (exemplified by SUV39H1 and EZH2/SUZ12) to promoters of E2F responsive proliferation genes leading to histone trimethylation and heterochromatin and thereby DAPI dense microscopic structures. Recent work indicates that H3K9 and H3K27, although usually associated with SAHF, may not be a strict requirement. Instead the formation of DAPI dense structures is linked to the timing of presenescent replication events [135]. This view would explain the fact that SWI/SNF including BRM has been associated in a transient manner with the build up of SAHF structures; BRM can also interact with pRb but strictly is associated with acetylated histones and replicating chromatin is acetylated [140]. The complete understanding of SAHF formation is still an evolving field. Regardless, it is widely accepted that functional p16^{INK4a} and pRb as well as the HMGA, which accumulate at E2F target promoters during senescence, are critically required for SAHF arrangement. In regards to p16^{INK4a} it is tempting to speculate that its specific role in SAHF formation goes beyond CDK inhibition and thus maintaining pRb in an active state.

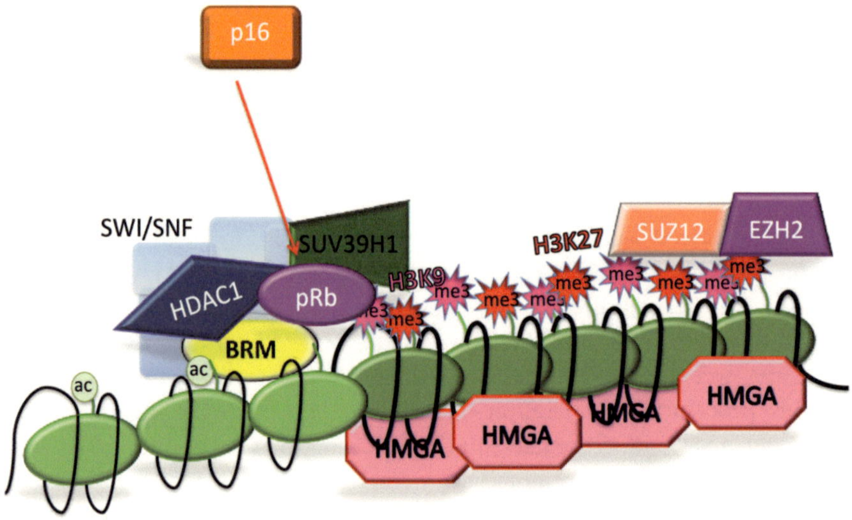

Figure 5. Chromatin remodeling and *SAHF formation*

8. Conclusion

Senescence is a potent means of tumor suppression. The mechanisms of senescence involve cell cycle regulatory protein functions in concert with the chromatin remodeling machinery to maintain a complex and secure withdrawal from proliferation. The understanding of these mechanisms is still evolving and is predicted to identify novel targets for cancer therapy.

Acknowledgements

We thank Dr Kavitha Gowrishankar for her assistance with the illustrations and Dr Roland Houben for the critical review of the manuscript.

http://dx.doi.org/10.5772/54120

Author details

Therese Becker[1] and Sebastian Haferkamp[2]

1 Westmead Institute for Cancer Research, University of Sydney at Westmead Millennium Institute, Westmead Hospital, Westmead, New South Wales, Australia

2 Department of Dermatology, Venereology und Allergology, University Hospital Würzburg, Germany

References

[1] De Cecco M, Jeyapalan J, Zhao X, Tamamori-Adachi M, Sedivy JM. Nuclear protein accumulation in cellular senescence and organismal aging revealed with a novel single-cell resolution fluorescence microscopy assay. Aging (Albany NY). 2011 Oct; 3(10):955-67.

[2] Dimri GP, Lee X, Basile G, Acosta M, Scott G, Roskelley C, et al. A biomarker that identifies senescent human cells in culture and in aging skin in vivo. Proc Natl Acad Sci U S A. 1995;92:9363-7.

[3] Lee BY, Han JA, Im JS, Morrone A, Johung K, Goodwin EC, et al. Senescence-associated beta-galactosidase is lysosomal beta-galactosidase. Aging Cell. 2006;5(2):187-95.

[4] Kurz DJ, Decary S, Hong Y, Erusalimsky JD. Senescence-associated (beta)-galactosidase reflects an increase in lysosomal mass during replicative ageing of human endothelial cells. J Cell Sci. 2000;113(Pt 20):3613-22.

[5] Severino J, Allen RG, Balin S, Balin A, Cristofalo VJ. Is beta-galactosidase staining a marker of senescence in vitro and in vivo? Exp Cell Res. 2000;257(1):162-71.

[6] Untergasser G, Gander R, Rumpold H, Heinrich E, Plas E, Berger P. TGF-beta cytokines increase senescence-associated beta-galactosidase activity in human prostate basal cells by supporting differentiation processes, but not cellular senescence. Exp Gerontol. 2003 Oct;38(10):1179-88.

[7] Yegorov YE, Akimov SS, Hass R, Zelenin AV, Prudovsky IA. Endogenous beta-galactosidase activity in continuously nonproliferating cells. Exp Cell Res. 1998 Aug 25;243(1):207-11.

[8] Cristofalo VJ. SA beta Gal staining: biomarker or delusion. Exp Gerontol. 2005 Oct; 40(10):836-8.

[9] Narita M, Nunez S, Heard E, Lin AW, Hearn SA, Spector DL, et al. Rb-mediated heterochromatin formation and silencing of E2F target genes during cellular senescence. Cell. 2003 Jun 13;113(6):703-16.

[10] Adams PD. Remodeling of chromatin structure in senescent cells and its potential impact on tumor suppression and aging. Gene. 2007 Aug 1;397(1-2):84-93.

[11] Weintraub SJ, Chow KN, Luo RX, Zhang SH, He S, Dean DC. Mechanism of active transcriptional repression by the retinoblastoma protein. Nature. 1995;375(6534): 812-5.

[12] Lavoie JN, L'Allemain G, Brunet A, Muller R, Pouyssegur J. Cyclin D1 expression is regulated positively by the p42/p44MAPK and negatively by the p38/HOGMAPK pathway. J Biol Chem. 1996 Aug 23;271(34):20608-16.

[13] Hanahan D, Weinberg RA. The hallmarks of cancer. Cell. 2000 Jan 7;100(1):57-70.

[14] Parry D, Mahony D, Wills K, Lees E. Cyclin D-CDK subunit arrangement is dependent on the availability of competing INK4 and p21 class inhibitors. Mol Cell Biol. 1999 Mar;19(3):1775-83.

[15] McConnell BB, Gregory FJ, Stott FJ, Hara E, Peters G. Induced expression of p16(INK4a) inhibits both CDK4- and CDK2-associated kinase activity by reassortment of cyclin-CDK-inhibitor complexes. Mol Cell Biol. 1999 Mar;19(3):1981-9.

[16] Hara E, Smith R, Parry D, Tahara H, Stone S, Peters G. Regulation of p16CDKN2 expression and its implications for cell immortalization and senescence. Mol Cell Biol. 1996 Mar;16(3):859-67.

[17] Alcorta DA, Xiong Y, Phelps D, Hannon G, Beach D, Barrett JC. Involvement of the cyclin-dependent kinase inhibitor p16 (INK4a) in replicative senescence of normal human fibroblasts. Proc Natl Acad Sci U S A. 1996 Nov 26;93(24):13742-7.

[18] Reznikoff CA, Yeager TR, Belair CD, Savelieva E, Puthenveettil JA, Stadler WM. Elevated p16 at senescence and loss of p16 at immortalization in human papillomavirus 16 E6, but not E7, transformed human uroepithelial cells. Cancer Res. 1996;56(13): 2886-90.

[19] Loughran O, Malliri A, Owens D, Gallimore PH, Stanley MA, Ozanne B, et al. Association of CDKN2A/p16INK4A with human head and neck keratinocyte replicative senescence: relationship of dysfunction to immortality and neoplasia. Oncogene. 1996 Aug 1;13(3):561-8.

[20] Erickson S, Sangfelt O, Heyman M, Castro J, Einhorn S, Grander D. Involvement of the Ink4 proteins p16 and p15 in T-lymphocyte senescence. Oncogene. 1998 Aug 6;17(5):595-602.

[21] Brenner AJ, Stampfer MR, Aldaz CM. Increased p16 expression with first senescence arrest in human mammary epithelial cells and extended growth capacity with p16 inactivation. Oncogene. 1998;17(2):199-205.

[22] Bandyopadhyay D, Medrano EE. Melanin accumulation accelerates melanocyte senescence by a mechanism involving p16INK4a/CDK4/pRB and E2F1. Ann N Y Acad Sci. 2000 Jun;908:71-84.

[23] Itahana K, Zou Y, Itahana Y, Martinez JL, Beausejour C, Jacobs JJ, et al. Control of the replicative life span of human fibroblasts by p16 and the polycomb protein Bmi-1. Mol Cell Biol. 2003 Jan;23(1):389-401.

[24] Noble JR, Rogan EM, Neumann AA, Maclean K, Bryan TM, Reddel RR. Association of extended in vitro proliferative potential with loss of p16INK4 expression. Oncogene. 1996 Sep 19;13(6):1259-68.

[25] Serrano M, Lin AW, McCurrach ME, Beach D, Lowe SW. Oncogenic ras provokes premature cell senescence associated with accumulation of p53 and p16INK4a. Cell. 1997 Mar 7;88(5):593-602.

[26] Zhu J, Woods D, McMahon M, Bishop JM. Senescence of human fibroblasts induced by oncogenic Raf. Genes Dev. 1998 Oct 1;12(19):2997-3007.

[27] Lin AW, Barradas M, Stone JC, van Aelst L, Serrano M, Lowe SW. Premature senescence involving p53 and p16 is activated in response to constitutive MEK/MAPK mitogenic signaling. Genes Dev. 1998 Oct 1;12(19):3008-19.

[28] Robles SJ, Adami GR. Agents that cause DNA double strand breaks lead to p16INK4a enrichment and the premature senescence of normal fibroblasts. Oncogene. 1998 Mar 5;16(9):1113-23.

[29] Michaloglou C, Vredeveld LC, Soengas MS, Denoyelle C, Kuilman T, van der Horst CM, et al. BRAFE600-associated senescence-like cell cycle arrest of human naevi. Nature. 2005;436(7051):720-4.

[30] te Poele RH, Okorokov AL, Jardine L, Cummings J, Joel SP. DNA damage is able to induce senescence in tumor cells in vitro and in vivo. Cancer Res. 2002 Mar 15;62(6): 1876-83.

[31] Ksiazek K, Mikula-Pietrasik J, Olijslagers S, Jorres A, von Zglinicki T, Witowski J. Vulnerability to oxidative stress and different patterns of senescence in human peritoneal mesothelial cell strains. Am J Physiol Regul Integr Comp Physiol. 2009 Feb; 296(2):R374-82.

[32] Klimova TA, Bell EL, Shroff EH, Weinberg FD, Snyder CM, Dimri GP, et al. Hyperoxia-induced premature senescence requires p53 and pRb, but not mitochondrial matrix ROS. FASEB J. 2009 Mar;23(3):783-94.

[33] Chen J, Patschan S, Goligorsky MS. Stress-induced premature senescence of endothelial cells. J Nephrol. 2008 May-Jun;21(3):337-44.

[34] Sharpless NE, Bardeesy N, Lee KH, Carrasco D, Castrillon DH, Aguirre AJ, et al. Loss of p16Ink4a with retention of p19Arf predisposes mice to tumorigenesis. Nature. 2001 Sep 6;413(6851):86-91.

[35] Krimpenfort P, Quon KC, Mooi WJ, Loonstra A, Berns A. Loss of p16Ink4a confers susceptibility to metastatic melanoma in mice. Nature. 2001 Sep 6;413(6851):83-6.

[36] Denoyelle C, Abou-Rjaily G, Bezrookove V, Verhaegen M, Johnson TM, Fullen DR, et al. Anti-oncogenic role of the endoplasmic reticulum differentially activated by mutations in the MAPK pathway. Nat Cell Biol. 2006 Oct;8(10):1053-63.

[37] Haferkamp S, Scurr LL, Becker TM, Frausto M, Kefford RF, Rizos H. Oncogene-Induced Senescence Does Not Require the p16(INK4a) or p14ARF Melanoma Tumor Suppressors. J Invest Dermatol. 2009 Feb 12.

[38] Beausejour CM, Krtolica A, Galimi F, Narita M, Lowe SW, Yaswen P, et al. Reversal of human cellular senescence: roles of the p53 and p16 pathways. EMBO J. 2003 Aug 15;22(16):4212-22.

[39] Kosar M, Bartkova J, Hubackova S, Hodny Z, Lukas J, Bartek J. Senescence-associated heterochromatin foci are dispensable for cellular senescence, occur in a cell type- and insult-dependent manner and follow expression of p16(ink4a). Cell Cycle. 2011 Feb 1;10(3):457-68.

[40] Di Micco R, Sulli G, Dobreva M, Liontos M, Botrugno OA, Gargiulo G, et al. Interplay between oncogene-induced DNA damage response and heterochromatin in senescence and cancer. Nat Cell Biol. 2011 Mar;13(3):292-302.

[41] Uhrbom L, Nister M, Westermark B. Induction of senescence in human malignant glioma cells by p16INK4A. Oncogene. 1997 Jul 31;15(5):505-14.

[42] Timmermann S, Hinds PW, Munger K. Re-expression of endogenous p16ink4a in oral squamous cell carcinoma lines by 5-aza-2'-deoxycytidine treatment induces a senescence-like state. Oncogene. 1998 Dec 31;17(26):3445-53.

[43] Dai CY, Enders GH. p16 INK4a can initiate an autonomous senescence program. Oncogene. 2000 Mar 23;19(13):1613-22.

[44] Becker TM, Rizos H, Kefford RF, Mann GJ. Functional impairment of melanoma-associated p16(INK4a) mutants in melanoma cells despite retention of cyclin-dependent kinase 4 binding. Clin Cancer Res. 2001 Oct;7(10):3282-8.

[45] Haferkamp S, Becker TM, Scurr LL, Kefford RF, Rizos H. p16INK4a-induced senescence is disabled by melanoma-associated mutations. Aging Cell. 2008 Oct;7(5): 733-45.

[46] McConnell BB, Starborg M, Brookes S, Peters G. Inhibitors of cyclin-dependent kinases induce features of replicative senescence in early passage human diploid fibroblasts. Curr Biol. 1998 Mar 12;8(6):351-4.

[47] Kato D, Miyazawa K, Ruas M, Starborg M, Wada I, Oka T, et al. Features of replicative senescence induced by direct addition of antennapedia-p16INK4A fusion protein to human diploid fibroblasts. FEBS Lett. 1998 May 8;427(2):203-8.

[48] Oguro H, Iwama A, Morita Y, Kamijo T, van Lohuizen M, Nakauchi H. Differential impact of Ink4a and Arf on hematopoietic stem cells and their bone marrow microenvironment in Bmi1-deficient mice. J Exp Med. 2006 Oct 2;203(10):2247-53.

[49] Molofsky AV, He S, Bydon M, Morrison SJ, Pardal R. Bmi-1 promotes neural stem cell self-renewal and neural development but not mouse growth and survival by repressing the p16Ink4a and p19Arf senescence pathways. Genes Dev. 2005 Jun 15;19(12):1432-7.

[50] Kotake Y, Cao R, Viatour P, Sage J, Zhang Y, Xiong Y. pRB family proteins are required for H3K27 trimethylation and Polycomb repression complexes binding to and silencing p16INK4alpha tumor suppressor gene. Genes Dev. 2007 Jan 1;21(1):49-54.

[51] Voncken JW, Niessen H, Neufeld B, Rennefahrt U, Dahlmans V, Kubben N, et al. MAPKAP kinase 3pK phosphorylates and regulates chromatin association of the polycomb group protein Bmi1. J Biol Chem. 2005 Feb 18;280(7):5178-87.

[52] Ohtani N, Zebedee Z, Huot TJ, Stinson JA, Sugimoto M, Ohashi Y, et al. Opposing effects of Ets and Id proteins on p16INK4a expression during cellular senescence. Nature. 2001;409(6823):1067-70.

[53] Yates PR, Atherton GT, Deed RW, Norton JD, Sharrocks AD. Id helix-loop-helix proteins inhibit nucleoprotein complex formation by the TCF ETS-domain transcription factors. EMBO J. 1999 Feb 15;18(4):968-76.

[54] Polsky D, Young AZ, Busam KJ, Alani RM. The transcriptional repressor of p16/Ink4a, Id1, is up-regulated in early melanomas. Cancer Res. 2001;61(16):6008-11.

[55] Zebedee Z, Hara E. Id proteins in cell cycle control and cellular senescence. Oncogene. 2001 Dec 20;20(58):8317-25.

[56] Cummings SD, Ryu B, Samuels MA, Yu X, Meeker AK, Healey MA, et al. Id1 delays senescence of primary human melanocytes. Mol Carcinog. 2008 Sep 1;47(9):653-9.

[57] Nickoloff BJ, Chaturvedi V, Bacon P, Qin JZ, Denning MF, Diaz MO. Id-1 delays senescence but does not immortalize keratinocytes. J Biol Chem. 2000 Sep 8;275(36):27501-4.

[58] Alani RM, Young AZ, Shifflett CB. Id1 regulation of cellular senescence through transcriptional repression of p16/Ink4a. Proc Natl Acad Sci U S A. 2001 Jul 3;98(14):7812-6.

[59] Lyden D, Young AZ, Zagzag D, Yan W, Gerald W, O'Reilly R, et al. Id1 and Id3 are required for neurogenesis, angiogenesis and vascularization of tumour xenografts. Nature. 1999 Oct 14;401(6754):670-7.

[60] Li M, Shin YH, Hou L, Huang X, Wei Z, Klann E, et al. The adaptor protein of the anaphase promoting complex Cdh1 is essential in maintaining replicative lifespan and in learning and memory. Nat Cell Biol. 2008 Sep;10(9):1083-9.

[61] Yang X, Sham JS, Ng MH, Tsao SW, Zhang D, Lowe SW, et al. LMP1 of Epstein-Barr virus induces proliferation of primary mouse embryonic fibroblasts and cooperatively transforms the cells with a p16-insensitive CDK4 oncogene. J Virol. 2000 Jan;74(2):883-91.

[62] Ohtani N, Brennan P, Gaubatz S, Sanij E, Hertzog P, Wolvetang E, et al. Epstein-Barr virus LMP1 blocks p16INK4a-RB pathway by promoting nuclear export of E2F4/5. J Cell Biol. 2003;162(2):173-83.

[63] Delmas V, Beermann F, Martinozzi S, Carreira S, Ackermann J, Kumasaka M, et al. Beta-catenin induces immortalization of melanocytes by suppressing p16INK4a expression and cooperates with N-Ras in melanoma development. Genes Dev. 2007;21(22):2923-35.

[64] Bachmann IM, Straume O, Puntervoll HE, Kalvenes MB, Akslen LA. Importance of P-cadherin, beta-catenin, and Wnt5a/frizzled for progression of melanocytic tumors and prognosis in cutaneous melanoma. Clin Cancer Res. 2005 Dec 15;11(24 Pt 1): 8606-14.

[65] Kageshita T, Hamby CV, Ishihara T, Matsumoto K, Saida T, Ono T. Loss of beta-catenin expression associated with disease progression in malignant melanoma. Br J Dermatol. 2001 Aug;145(2):210-6.

[66] Arozarena I, Bischof H, Gilby D, Belloni B, Dummer R, Wellbrock C. In melanoma, beta-catenin is a suppressor of invasion. Oncogene. 2011 Nov 10;30(45):4531-43.

[67] Gray-Schopfer VC, Cheong SC, Chong H, Chow J, Moss T, Abdel-Malek ZA, et al. Cellular senescence in naevi and immortalisation in melanoma: a role for p16? Br J Cancer. 2006 Aug 21;95(4):496-505.

[68] Tran SL, Haferkamp S, Scurr LL, Gowrishankar K, Becker TM, Desilva C, et al. Absence of distinguishing senescence traits in human melanocytic nevi. J Invest Dermatol. Sep;132(9):2226-34.

[69] Jacobs JJ, Keblusek P, Robanus-Maandag E, Kristel P, Lingbeek M, Nederlof PM, et al. Senescence bypass screen identifies TBX2, which represses Cdkn2a (p19(ARF)) and is amplified in a subset of human breast cancers. Nat Genet. 2000 Nov;26(3): 291-9.

[70] Vance KW, Carreira S, Brosch G, Goding CR. Tbx2 is overexpressed and plays an important role in maintaining proliferation and suppression of senescence in melanomas. Cancer Res. 2005 Mar 15;65(6):2260-8.

[71] Kia SK, Gorski MM, Giannakopoulos S, Verrijzer CP. SWI/SNF mediates polycomb eviction and epigenetic reprogramming of the INK4b-ARF-INK4a locus. Mol Cell Biol. 2008 May;28(10):3457-64.

[72] Betz BL, Strobeck MW, Reisman DN, Knudsen ES, Weissman BE. Re-expression of hSNF5/INI1/BAF47 in pediatric tumor cells leads to G1 arrest associated with induction of p16ink4a and activation of RB. Oncogene. 2002 Aug 8;21(34):5193-203.

[73] Oruetxebarria I, Venturini F, Kekarainen T, Houweling A, Zuijderduijn LM, Mohd-Sarip A, et al. P16INK4a is required for hSNF5 chromatin remodeler-induced cellular senescence in malignant rhabdoid tumor cells. J Biol Chem. 2004;279(5):3807-16. Epub 2003 Nov 06.

[74] Huot TJ, Rowe J, Harland M, Drayton S, Brookes S, Gooptu C, et al. Biallelic mutations in p16(INK4a) confer resistance to Ras- and Ets-induced senescence in human diploid fibroblasts. Mol Cell Biol. 2002 Dec;22(23):8135-43.

[75] Leong WF, Chau JF, Li B. p53 Deficiency leads to compensatory up-regulation of p16INK4a. Mol Cancer Res. 2009 Mar;7(3):354-60.

[76] Fujikawa M, Katagiri T, Tugores A, Nakamura Y, Ishikawa F. ESE-3, an Ets family transcription factor, is up-regulated in cellular senescence. Cancer Sci. 2007 Sep;98(9): 1468-75.

[77] Wu J, Xue L, Weng M, Sun Y, Zhang Z, Wang W, et al. Sp1 is essential for p16 expression in human diploid fibroblasts during senescence. PLoS ONE. 2007;2(1):e164.

[78] Wang X, Pan L, Feng Y, Wang Y, Han Q, Han L, et al. P300 plays a role in p16(INK4a) expression and cell cycle arrest. Oncogene. 2008 Mar 20;27(13):1894-904.

[79] Rubbi CP, Milner J. Disruption of the nucleolus mediates stabilization of p53 in response to DNA damage and other stresses. EMBO J. 2003;22:6068-77.

[80] Haupt Y, Maya R, Kaza A, Oren M. Mdm2 promotes the rapid degradation of p53. Nature. 1997;387:296-9.

[81] Lee JT, Gu W. The multiple levels of regulation by p53 ubiquitination. Cell Death Differ. 2010 Jan;17(1):86-92.

[82] Wang Y, Blandino G, Oren M, Givol D. Induced p53 expression in lung cancer cell line promotes cell senescence and differentially modifies the cytotoxicity of anti-cancer drugs. Oncogene. 1998 Oct 15;17(15):1923-30.

[83] Brown JP, Wei W, Sedivy JM. Bypass of senescence after disruption of p21CIP1/WAF1 gene in normal diploid human fibroblasts. Science. 1997;277(5327):831-4.

[84] Stott FJ, Bates S, James MC, McConnell BB, Starborg M, Brookes S, et al. The alternative product from the human CDKN2A locus, $p14^{ARF}$, participates in a regulatory feedback loop with p53 and MDM2. EMBO J. 1998;17(17):5001-14.

[85] Fang L, Igarashi M, Leung J, Sugrue MM, Lee SW, Aaronson SA. p21Waf1/Cip1/Sdi1 induces permanent growth arrest with markers of replicative senescence in human tumor cells lacking functional p53. Oncogene. 1999 May 6;18(18):2789-97.

[86] Wang Y, Blandino G, Givol D. Induced p21waf expression in H1299 cell line promotes cell senescence and protects against cytotoxic effect of radiation and doxorubicin. Oncogene. 1999 Apr 22;18(16):2643-9.

[87] Wei W, Hemmer RM, Sedivy JM. Role of p14(ARF) in replicative and induced senescence of human fibroblasts. Mol Cell Biol. 2001 Oct;21(20):6748-57.

[88] Villalonga-Planells R, Coll-Mulet L, Martinez-Soler F, Castano E, Acebes JJ, Gimenez-Bonafe P, et al. Activation of p53 by nutlin-3a induces apoptosis and cellular senescence in human glioblastoma multiforme. PLoS One. 2011;6(4):e18588.

[89] Harvey DM, Levine AJ. p53 alteration is a common event in the spontaneous immortalization of primary BALB/c murine embryo fibroblasts. Genes Dev. 1991 Dec; 5(12B):2375-85.

[90] Kamijo T, Zindy F, Roussel MF, Quelle DE, Downing JR, Ashmun RA, et al. Tumor suppression at the mouse INK4a locus mediated by the alternative reading frame product $p19^{ARF}$. Cell. 1997;91:649-59.

[91] Kamijo T, van de Kamp E, Chong MJ, Zindy F, Diehl JA, Sherr CJ, et al. Loss of the ARF tumor suppressor reverses premature replicative arrest but not radiation hypersensitivity arising from disabled atm function. Cancer Res. 1999 May 15;59(10): 2464-9.

[92] Gire V, Wynford-Thomas D. Reinitiation of DNA synthesis and cell division in senescent human fibroblasts by microinjection of anti-p53 antibodies. Mol Cell Biol. 1998 Mar;18(3):1611-21.

[93] Hara E, Tsurui H, Shinozaki A, Nakada S, Oda K. Cooperative effect of antisense-Rb and antisense-p53 oligomers on the extension of life span in human diploid fibroblasts, TIG-1. Biochem Biophys Res Commun. 1991 Aug 30;179(1):528-34.

[94] Shay JW, Pereira-Smith OM, Wright WE. A role for both RB and p53 in the regulation of human cellular senescence. Exp Cell Res. 1991 Sep;196(1):33-9.

[95] Sakamoto K, Howard T, Ogryzko V, Xu NZ, Corsico CC, Jones DH, et al. Relative mitogenic activities of wild-type and retinoblastoma binding-defective SV40 T antigens in serum-deprived and senescent human diploid fibroblasts. Oncogene. 1993 Jul;8(7):1887-93.

[96] Herbig U, Jobling WA, Chen BP, Chen DJ, Sedivy JM. Telomere shortening triggers senescence of human cells through a pathway involving ATM, p53, and p21(CIP1), but not p16(INK4a). Mol Cell. 2004;14(4):501-13.

[97] Haferkamp S, Tran SL, Becker TM, Scurr LL, Kefford RF, Rizos H. The relative contributions of the p53 and pRb pathways in oncogene-induced melanocyte senescence. Aging (Albany NY). 2009 Jun;1(6):542-56.

[98] Demidenko ZN, Korotchkina LG, Gudkov AV, Blagosklonny MV. Paradoxical suppression of cellular senescence by p53. Proc Natl Acad Sci U S A. 2010 May 25;107(21):9660-4.

[99] Demidenko ZN, Blagosklonny MV. Growth stimulation leads to cellular senescence when the cell cycle is blocked. Cell Cycle. 2008 Nov 1;7(21):3355-61.

[100] Demidenko ZN, Zubova SG, Bukreeva EI, Pospelov VA, Pospelova TV, Blagosklonny MV. Rapamycin decelerates cellular senescence. Cell Cycle. 2009 Jun 15;8(12): 1888-95.

[101] Demidenko ZN, Blagosklonny MV. Quantifying pharmacologic suppression of cellular senescence: prevention of cellular hypertrophy versus preservation of proliferative potential. Aging (Albany NY). 2009 Dec;1(12):1008-16.

[102] Maser RS, Monsen KJ, Nelms BE, Petrini JH. hMre11 and hRad50 nuclear foci are induced during the normal cellular response to DNA double-strand breaks. Mol Cell Biol. 1997 Oct;17(10):6087-96.

[103] de Jager M, Dronkert ML, Modesti M, Beerens CE, Kanaar R, van Gent DC. DNA-binding and strand-annealing activities of human Mre11: implications for its roles in DNA double-strand break repair pathways. Nucleic Acids Res. 2001 Mar 15;29(6): 1317-25.

[104] de Jager M, van Noort J, van Gent DC, Dekker C, Kanaar R, Wyman C. Human Rad50/Mre11 is a flexible complex that can tether DNA ends. Mol Cell. 2001 Nov; 8(5):1129-35.

[105] Paull TT, Gellert M. Nbs1 potentiates ATP-driven DNA unwinding and endonuclease cleavage by the Mre11/Rad50 complex. Genes Dev. 1999 May 15;13(10): 1276-88.

[106] Paull TT, Lee JH. The Mre11/Rad50/Nbs1 complex and its role as a DNA double-strand break sensor for ATM. Cell Cycle. 2005 Jun;4(6):737-40.

[107] Trujillo KM, Sung P. DNA structure-specific nuclease activities in the Saccharomyces cerevisiae Rad50*Mre11 complex. J Biol Chem. 2001 Sep 21;276(38):35458-64.

[108] Sancar A, Lindsey-Boltz LA, Unsal-Kacmaz K, Linn S. Molecular mechanisms of mammalian DNA repair and the DNA damage checkpoints. Annu Rev Biochem. 2004;73:39-85.

[109] Collado M, Blasco MA, Serrano M. Cellular senescence in cancer and aging. Cell. 2007 Jul 27;130(2):223-33.

[110] Sherr CJ, McCormick F. The RB and p53 pathways in cancer. Cancer Cell. 2002;2(2): 103-12.

[111] Chang BD, Broude EV, Dokmanovic M, Zhu H, Ruth A, Xuan Y, et al. A senescence-like phenotype distinguishes tumor cells that undergo terminal proliferation arrest after exposure to anticancer agents. Cancer Res. 1999 Aug 1;59(15):3761-7.

[112] Wang X, Wong SC, Pan J, Tsao SW, Fung KH, Kwong DL, et al. Evidence of cisplatin-induced senescent-like growth arrest in nasopharyngeal carcinoma cells. Cancer Res. 1998 Nov 15;58(22):5019-22.

[113] Yeo EJ, Hwang YC, Kang CM, Kim IH, Kim DI, Parka JS, et al. Senescence-like changes induced by hydroxyurea in human diploid fibroblasts. Exp Gerontol. 2000 Aug;35(5):553-71.

[114] Michishita E, Nakabayashi K, Suzuki T, Kaul SC, Ogino H, Fujii M, et al. 5-Bromodeoxyuridine induces senescence-like phenomena in mammalian cells regardless of cell type or species. J Biochem. 1999 Dec;126(6):1052-9.

[115] Chen QM. Replicative senescence and oxidant-induced premature senescence. Beyond the control of cell cycle checkpoints. Ann N Y Acad Sci. 2000 Jun;908:111-25.

[116] Jackson JG, Pant V, Li Q, Chang LL, Quintas-Cardama A, Garza D, et al. p53-mediated senescence impairs the apoptotic response to chemotherapy and clinical outcome in breast cancer. Cancer Cell. 2012 Jun 12;21(6):793-806.

[117] Lu T, Finkel T. Free radicals and senescence. Exp Cell Res. 2008 Jun 10;314(9):1918-22.

[118] Fang K, Chiu CC, Li CH, Chang YT, Hwang HT. Cisplatin-induced senescence and growth inhibition in human non-small cell lung cancer cells with ectopic transfer of p16INK4a. Oncol Res. 2007;16(10):479-88.

[119] Schmitt CA, Fridman JS, Yang M, Lee S, Baranov E, Hoffman RM, et al. A senescence program controlled by p53 and p16INK4a contributes to the outcome of cancer therapy. Cell. 2002;109(3):335-46.

[120] Moiseeva O, Mallette FA, Mukhopadhyay UK, Moores A, Ferbeyre G. DNA damage signaling and p53-dependent senescence after prolonged beta-interferon stimulation. Mol Biol Cell. 2006 Apr;17(4):1583-92.

[121] Elmore LW, Rehder CW, Di X, McChesney PA, Jackson-Cook CK, Gewirtz DA, et al. Adriamycin-induced senescence in breast tumor cells involves functional p53 and telomere dysfunction. J Biol Chem. 2002 Sep 20;277(38):35509-15.

[122] Duan J, Zhang Z, Tong T. Irreversible cellular senescence induced by prolonged exposure to H2O2 involves DNA-damage-and-repair genes and telomere shortening. Int J Biochem Cell Biol. 2005 Jul;37(7):1407-20.

[123] Berndtsson M, Hagg M, Panaretakis T, Havelka AM, Shoshan MC, Linder S. Acute apoptosis by cisplatin requires induction of reactive oxygen species but is not associated with damage to nuclear DNA. Int J Cancer. 2007 Jan 1;120(1):175-80.

[124] Zhao W, Lin ZX, Zhang ZQ. Cisplatin-induced premature senescence with concomitant reduction of gap junctions in human fibroblasts. Cell Res. 2004 Feb;14(1):60-6.

[125] Duale N, Lindeman B, Komada M, Olsen AK, Andreassen A, Soderlund EJ, et al. Molecular portrait of cisplatin induced response in human testis cancer cell lines based on gene expression profiles. Mol Cancer. 2007;6:53.

[126] Di Micco R, Fumagalli M, Cicalese A, Piccinin S, Gasparini P, Luise C, et al. Oncogene-induced senescence is a DNA damage response triggered by DNA hyper-replication. Nature. 2006 Nov 30;444(7119):638-42.

[127] Bartkova J, Rezaei N, Liontos M, Karakaidos P, Kletsas D, Issaeva N, et al. Oncogene-induced senescence is part of the tumorigenesis barrier imposed by DNA damage checkpoints. Nature. 2006 Nov 30;444(7119):633-7.

[128] Xu HJ, Zhou Y, Ji W, Perng GS, Kruzelock R, Kong CT, et al. Reexpression of the retinoblastoma protein in tumor cells induces senescence and telomerase inhibition. Oncogene. 1997 Nov 20;15(21):2589-96.

[129] Becker TM. Chromatin Remodeling in Carcinoma Cells. In: Meyers RA, editor. Encyclopedia of Molecular Cell Biology and Molecular Medicine: Wiley-VCH Verlag GmbH & Co. KGaA; 2012. p. 973-1007.

[130] Ferreira R, Naguibneva I, Mathieu M, Ait-Si-Ali S, Robin P, Pritchard LL, et al. Cell cycle-dependent recruitment of HDAC-1 correlates with deacetylation of histone H4 on an Rb-E2F target promoter. EMBO Rep. 2001 Sep;2(9):794-9.

[131] Funayama R, Ishikawa F. Cellular senescence and chromatin structure. Chromosoma. 2007 Oct;116(5):431-40.

[132] Nielsen SJ, Schneider R, Bauer UM, Bannister AJ, Morrison A, O'Carroll D, et al. Rb targets histone H3 methylation and HP1 to promoters. Nature. 2001 Aug 2;412(6846): 561-5.

[133] Kim KC, Geng L, Huang S. Inactivation of a histone methyltransferase by mutations in human cancers. Cancer Res. 2003 Nov 15;63(22):7619-23.

[134] Cloos PA, Christensen J, Agger K, Maiolica A, Rappsilber J, Antal T, et al. The putative oncogene GASC1 demethylates tri- and dimethylated lysine 9 on histone H3. Nature. 2006 Jul 20;442(7100):307-11.

[135] Chandra T, Kirschner K, Thuret JY, Pope BD, Ryba T, Newman S, et al. Independence of Repressive Histone Marks and Chromatin Compaction during Senescent Heterochromatic Layer Formation. Mol Cell. 2012 Jul 27;47(2):203-14.

[136] Bandyopadhyay D, Okan NA, Bales E, Nascimento L, Cole PA, Medrano EE. Down-regulation of p300/CBP histone acetyltransferase activates a senescence checkpoint in human melanocytes. Cancer Res. 2002 Nov 1;62(21):6231-9.

[137] Zhang HS, Gavin M, Dahiya A, Postigo AA, Ma D, Luo RX, et al. Exit from G1 and S phase of the cell cycle is regulated by repressor complexes containing HDAC-Rb-hSWI/SNF and Rb-hSWI/SNF. Cell. 2000 Mar 31;101(1):79-89.

[138] Kang H, Cui K, Zhao K. BRG1 controls the activity of the retinoblastoma protein via regulation of p21CIP1/WAF1/SDI. Mol Cell Biol. 2004 Feb;24(3):1188-99.

[139] Becker TM, Haferkamp S, Dijkstra MK, Scurr LL, Frausto M, Diefenbach E, et al. The chromatin remodelling factor BRG1 is a novel binding partner of the tumor suppressor p16INK4a. Mol Cancer. 2009;8:4.

[140] Bandyopadhyay D, Curry JL, Lin Q, Richards HW, Chen D, Hornsby PJ, et al. Dynamic assembly of chromatin complexes during cellular senescence: implications for the growth arrest of human melanocytic nevi. Aging Cell. 2007 Aug;6(4):577-91.

[141] Haferkamp S, Scurr LL, Becker TM, Frausto M, Kefford RF, Rizos H. Oncogene-induced senescence does not require the p16(INK4a) or p14ARF melanoma tumor suppressors. J Invest Dermatol. 2009 Aug;129(8):1983-91.

Section 3

Plant Senescence

Chapter 3

Plant Senescence and Nitrogen Mobilization and Signaling

Stefan Bieker and Ulrike Zentgraf

Additional information is available at the end of the chapter

http://dx.doi.org/10.5772/54392

1. Introduction

1.1. Senescence

Very early during their reproductive phase, annual plants initiate the process of senescence. Monocarpic senescence describes the last steps in these plants' development; senescence on organ level starts shortly after entering reproductive phase while after anthesis the whole plant undergoes senescence and dies.

In the following we will focus on leaf senescence. Two different processes can be distinguished in annual plants relying on different genetic programs. Before anthesis, sequential leaf senescence recycles nutrients from old to developing leaves which is mainly under the control of the growing apex and is arrested when no more new leaves develop and when the plant starts to flower and sets fruit. Monocarpic leaf senescence recovers valuable nutrients from the leaves during flower induction and anthesis to provide these to the developing reproductive organs [1, 2]. The latter is crucial for fruit and seed development and has a major impact on yield quantity and quality. In wheat salvaged nitrogen (N) from the leaves accounts for up to 90% of the total grain N content [3]. A complex regulation of many different metabolic pathways and expression of numerous genes underlies this process. How coordination and interplay of many controlling factors, like hormones, genetic reprogramming, biotic and abiotic stresses are achieved is far from being understood, but it is already clear that this regulatory network is highly complex and dynamic.

Thousands of genes are differentially regulated during senescence induction and progression. To date forward and reverse genetic approaches as well as large-scale transcript profiling have identified almost 6.500 genes being differentially expressed during the course of leaf senescence including up-regulated as well as down-regulated genes [4]. The high number of differentially regulated senescence-associated transcription factors (TF) demonstrates the dimensions of genetic reprogramming taking place. These TFs include 20 distinct families of which NAC-, WRKY-, C2H2-type zinc finger, EREBP- and MYB-families are most abundant [5]. Recently, Breeze et al. (2011) [4] published extremely important results of a high-resolution temporal transcript profiling of senescing Arabidopsis leaves giving insight into the temporal order of genetic events. One of the first steps at the onset of senescence is a shift from anabolic to catabolic processes. Amino acid metabolism and protein synthesis are down-regulated while expression of autophagy- and reactive oxygen species-related, and water-response genes is enhanced. In contrast to the following elevation of abscisic acid (ABA) and jasmonic acid (JA) signaling-related gene expression, cytokinin-mediated signaling is lowered just as chlorophyll and carotenoid biosynthesis. The next phases include down-regulation of carbon utilization and enhanced expression of cystein-aspartat proteases, carotene metabolism-associated genes and pectinesterases which is then followed by the reduction of photosynthetic activity and degradation of the photosynthetic apparatus coinciding with the increased activity of lipid catabolism, ethylene signaling and higher abundance of cytoskeletal elements [4].

Hormonal control of senescence is conveyed especially by ethylene, jasmonic and salicylic acid, cytokinin and auxin. Many mutants with a delayed senescence phenotype could be traced back to impaired or up-regulated ethylene or cytokinin signaling, respectively [6, 7]. In adition, ABA acts as a positive regulator of leaf senescence. Recently a membrane-bound, leucine rich repeat containing receptor kinase (RPK1) has been identified to play an important role in ABA-mediated senescence induction in an age-dependent manner. Strikingly, *rpk1* mutant lines did not show significant alterations in developmental processes, which have been reported for numerous other ABA signaling defective mutant lines [5], except slightly shorter growth [8]. This kinase has been indentified to integrate ABA signals during seed germination, plant growth, stomatal closure and stress responses. Overexpression lines showed enhanced expression of several stress and H_2O_2-responsive genes [9, 10]. Mutant lines showed a delayed senescence phenotype with slower progression of chlorophyll degradation and cell death.

Induction and progression of leaf senescence demands a tight regulation of numerous processes. Integration of nutritional cues, biotic and abiotic influences, plant development and age has to take place for the correct timing of onset and temporal advance of this complex developmental process. Despite the enormous efforts and achievements in this field, many of the regulatory mechanisms remain elusive.

1.2. Nitrogen and agriculture

The nowadays growth of population and thus increasing demand for food and oil crops forces agricultural industry to increase quantitative as well as qualitative yields. Until 2050 world's population is predicted to be as high as 9-10 billion people [11] and grain requirement is projected to be doubled, mostly resulting from a higher demand for wheat fed meat [12]. As most of the cropping systems are naturally deficient in nitrogen, there is a fundamental dependency on inorganic nitrogen fertilizers. 85-90 million tons of these fertilizers are applied annually worldwide [13-15]. However, 50-70% of these nitrogenous fertilizer are lost to the environment [16], mostly due to volatilization of N_2O, NO, N_2 and NH_3 and leaching of soluble NO_3^- into the water. Thus nitrogen is not only one of the most expensive nutrients to provide, but it also has a strong detrimental impact on the environment. Since surrounding ecosystems and potable water supply are endangered by oversaturation with nitrogenous compounds, it is necessary to improve application techniques and plant's nitrogen use efficiencies.

Several different definitions of nitrogen and nutrient use efficiencies are on hand. The most common is the *nitrogen use efficiency* (NUE), which is defined as shoot dry weight divided by total nitrogen content of the shoots. The *usage index* (UI) takes absolute biomass into account as it is denoted by the shoot fresh weight times the NUE. Likewise, the *N uptake efficiency* (NUpE) takes into account the whole N content of the plant and the N supplied by fertilization per plant. The fraction of the N taken up, which is then distributed to the grain, can be obtained by calculating the *N utilization efficiency* (NUtE) (Grain weight per total N content). Other efficiencies, which seem to be more suitable for the use in applied sciences, are the *agronomic efficiency* (AE), *apparent nitrogen recovery* (AR) and the *physiological efficiency* (PE). AE, AR and PE do require an unfertilized control to be calculated. While AE measures the efficiency to redirect applied nitrogen to the grains, AR defines the efficiency to capture N from the soil. PE puts the N uptake into relationship with the outcome of grain (reviewed in [15]). *Nitrogen remobilization efficiency* (NRE) describes the plant's capacity to translocate already assimilated nitrogen to developing organs. Finally, the *harvest index* (HI) and the *nitrogen harvest index* (NHI) are often used terms. HI is the total yield weight per plant mass, while NHI states the grain N content per whole plant N content.

Emission of nitrogen to the environment could be strongly reduced by application of 'best management techniques' in agricultural practice like e.g. rectifying the rate of appliance by accounting for all other possible sources of nitrogen influx (carryover from previous crops, atmospheric deposits etc.), ameliorating the timing and also changing the method of appliance to reduce atmospheric losses [13]. Food production has doubled in the last 40 years. Most of this increase could be achieved by selection of new strains, breeding and application of greater amounts of fertilizer and pesticides and other techniques [12]. Amending of nutrient use efficiencies of the crop plants was mostly accomplished via breeding programs by now. QTL selection for higher yields, increased oil or protein content has been pursued for decades. In wheat for example, increasing yield and grain protein content has been extensively studied, but improving both is restrained by the negative genetic relationship between these traits [17, 18].

2. Nitrogen uptake, assimilation and distribution

Nitrogen sources vary extremely encompassing organic and inorganic forms, small peptides and single amino acids, thus uptake systems need to be adjusted and well regulated in spatial and temporal activity. Although the predominant form in which N is taken up mainly depends on the plants adaption to the given environment and influences like fertilization, soil pH, temperature, precipitation and others [14, 19], most plants cover their N demand primarily through soil nitrate being provided by fertilization, bacterial nitrification and other processes [15]. However, a wide range of different uptake system has evolved in plants. For example, oligopeptides can be taken up via OPT-proteins (oligopeptide transporters), ammonium via ammonium transporters (AMTs) and amino acids via amino acid transporters and amino acid permeases. Besides the *AtCLC* (ChLoride Channel) gene family, comprising 7 members of which two (*AtCLCa* and *AtCLCb*) have been shown to encode tonoplast located NO_3^-/H^+ antiporters [20, 21], two families of nitrate transporters have been identified in higher plants (NRT1 and NRT2), representing low- and high affinity transporter systems, respectively. Moreover the *NRT1*-family has been shown to comprise also di-/tripeptide transporters (PTR) [22].

2.1. Nitrogen transporter systems

Four constituents of nitrate uptake are known, constitutive (c) and inducible (i) high- (HAT) and low-affinity (LAT) transporters, respectively. The high-affinity system's K_M ranges from ~ 5-100 μM, varying with plant species, and a maximal influx via this system of 1 $\mu Mol * g^{-1} * h^{-1}$ has been determined [23, 24]. At nitrate concentrations of 10 mM the influx rate via the LATs can reach up to ~24 $\mu Mol * g^{-1} * h^{-1}$ [24].

The *NRT1*-family comprises 53 genes in Arabidopsis which are classified as LATs. *AtNRT1-1 (CHL1)* was the first member to be identified in 1993 and has been shown to encode a proton-coupled nitrate transporter [25]. Studies with *Xenopus* oocytes have shown that this transporter protein possesses two different states, one serving low-affinity and the other one high-affinity nitrate uptake [26, 27], thus the distinction between high and low-affinity nitrate transporters is overridden in this case. Switching between these two modes of action is conferred by phosphorylation of threonin at position 101 [28]. *AtNRT1-1* is expressed in the cortex and endodermis of mature roots and in the epidermis of root tips. Additionally, a nitrate sensing function regulating the plants primary nitrate response has been strongly indicated for the AtNRT1-1 protein by several lines of evidence. The *chl1-5 (atnrt1-1-5)* mutant, a deletion mutant with no detectable *CHL1* transcript, is deficient in nitrate uptake and initiation of the primary nitrate response. The *chl1-9* mutant is defective in nitrate uptake but not in the primary nitrate response. The *chl1-9* mutant has a point mutation between two transmembrane domains. When threonine 101 was mutated to mimic or repress phosphorylation and transformed into the *chl1-5* background, primary nitrate response could be repressed or enhanced [29]. Constitutive expression identifies AtNRT1-2 as part of the Arabidopsis cLATs. Its transcript is only found in root epidermal cells [22]. Expression of *AtNRT1-5* is nitrate inducible; however, the response to nitrate is much slower than for *AtNRT1-1*. AtNRT1-5 has been shown to be a pH-dependent, bidirectional nitrate transporter, with subcellular localization in the plasma membrane of root pericycle cells near the xylem implicating an involvement in long-distance nitrate transport [30]. Experimental evidence suggests nitrate storage in leaf petioles to be associated with the function of AtNRT1-4. Here, nitrate content is relatively high, while nitrate reductase (NR) activity is low. Additionally, *AtNRT1-4* is predominantly expressed in the leaf petiole and the *atnrt1.4* mutant shows a nitrate content decreased by half in the petiole [22, 31]. *AtNRT1-6* is expressed in the silique's and funiculus' vascular tissue and thought to play a nitrate providing role in early embryonic development [32]. AtNRT1-8 functions in nitrate unloading from the xylem sap and is mainly located in xylem parenchyma cells within the vasculature [33], whereas AtNRT1-9 facilitates nitrate loading into the root phloem from root phloem companion cells [34].

High affinity nitrate uptake is conducted by members of the *NRT2*-family, comprising 7 genes in Arabidopsis. AtNRT2-1 has been shown to be one of the main components of the HATs. Mutant *atnrt2-1* plants displayed a loss of nitrate uptake capacity up to 75% at HAT-specific NO_3^- concentrations [35]. Furthermore, lateral root growth is repressed under low nitrate combined with high sucrose supply, where NRT2-1 acts either as sensor or transducer [36]. Experiments with *Xenopus* oocytes revealed the requirement of a AtNAR2 protein for AtNRT2-1 function [37]. Mutants of either of these two components showed impaired nitrate uptake at HAT-specific concentrations and hampered growth with display of N-starvation symptoms, in which, remarkably, the *atnar2* mutant phenotype appeared to be more pronounced [38]. The phenotype of the *atnrt2-7* mutant is similar to the phenotype of the *atclca* mutant. The *AtCLCa* gene has been shown to encode a NO_3^-/H^+ antiporter enabling accumulation of nitrate in the vacuole. Mutation of either of these resulted in lower nitrate content. Ectopic overexpression of *AtNRT2-7* led to higher nitrate contents in dried seeds, where the gene is highly expressed under wild type conditions, and an increase in the nitrate HATs uptake capacity by 2-fold. However, normal development was not impaired in the mutants as well as overexpressor plants [14, 20, 39]. Despite its high homology to *AtNRT2-1, AtNRT2-4* is not dependent on the function of *AtNAR2*. *AtNRT2-4* expression is highly induced upon nitrogen starvation in the outermost layer of young lateral roots [40].

Members of the *AMT1*- and *AMT2*-subfamilies are thought to be the main high affinity ammonium transporters in plants. Due to ammonium's toxic nature and convertibility from NH_4^+ to NH_3 and the thus varying membrane permeability, its uptake and transport needs to be tightly regulated [41, 42]. AMTs are regulated transcriptionally by N-supply, sugar and daytime and provide an additive contribution to ammonium transport [41]. AtAMT1-1 contributes 30-35 % as does AtAMT1-3, while AtAMT1-2 provides only 18-25% [43, 44]. AtAMT1-1 transports ammonium as well as its analog methyl-ammonium. Additionally, its activity is regulated posttranscriptionally via the availability of nitrate [42].

2.2. Nitrogen assimilation

Assimilation of NO_3^- and NH_4^+ almost always includes incorporation into amino acids (AA). The most abundant transport forms are glutamine, glutamate, asparagine and aspartate [45] although direct transport of NO_3^- and NH_4^+ also takes place but to a much lesser extend [46]. Nitrate assimilation thus requires reduction to ammonium. Nitrate reductase (NR) realizes the first step by reducing NO_3^- to NO_2^-. This reaction takes place in the cytoplasm, while the reduction of nitrite to ammonium is carried out in the plastids. Here, nitrite reductase (NiR) converts NO_2^- to NH_4^+ making it readily available for the incorporation into AAs in a NADH-dependent manner. Assimilation of ammonium into AAs involves chloroplastic glutamine synthetase 2 (GS2) and glutamate synthase (Fd-GOGAT), which generates glutamine and glutamate (for detailed review see [14]). Glutamine as well as glutamate serve as ammonium donor for the synthesis of all other amino acids including aspartate and asparagine, which in turn function as active NH_4^+ donor or as long-range nitrogen transport and storage form, respectively [47]. Alternatively carbamoylphosphate synthase can be involved in ammonium assimilation by producing carbamoylphosphate and successively citrulline and arginine. Assimilation in non-green tissues is achieved in plastids in a similar manner, although here GOGAT depends on NADH instead of ferredoxin. Carbon skeletons are essential for the acquisition of inorganic nitrogen in AAs. Especially the demand for keto-acids has to be met (see [14] and references within). These are predominantly obtained from the TCA-Cycle in the form of 2-oxoglutarate (2OG) [47, 48]. 2OG is used for incorporation of photorespiratory ammonium, resulting in the production of glutamate, which in turn can be utilized by GS1 and GS2 to produce glutamine. This displays the intricate interconnection between carbon and nitrogen metabolism, in which N uptake and assimilation is also influenced via photosynthetic rates [47]. Besides direct assimilation into AAs, nitrate can also be stored in the vacuole and in the chloroplast. Vacuolar nitrate concentrations can vary enormously, as vacuolar nitrate also contributes to turgor maintenance and might have a nitrate storage function to maintain the cytosolic nitrate concentrations which are more constant [49].

3. Senescence induction and nitrogen mobilization

As mentioned above, induction of senescence is a highly complex regulated and dynamic process. Besides developmental cues, there are numerous other possible impacts. Nutritional starvation, photosynthetic activity, pathogen infections, carbon accumulation, carbon to nitrogen ratio, photoperiod and various other cues can lead to senescence induction on either organ or whole plant level. Both natural and stress induced senescence are accompanied with the remobilization of valuable nutrients from various organs of the plant. In the following we will again focus on the situation in leaves.

3.1. Senescence induction

Correct timing of leaf senescence is crucial for proper plant development. Too early senescence induction would decrease the ability to assimilate CO_2, while too late induction would reduce the plant's capacity to remobilize nutrients from old leaves to developing organs [50]. Nevertheless, timing of senescence can also be regarded as an active adaption to the given nutritional and environmental conditions. For example under limited nutrition, continued growth of vegetative tissues would result in a reduced ability to develop reproductive organs.

Nutritional limitation, especially in concerns of nitrogen, has been shown to be able to enhance leaf senescence. Sunflower (*Helianthus annuus*) plants grown under low nitrogen supply showed a stronger decline of photosynthetic activity and more pronounced senescence symptoms than plants sufficiently supplied with nitrogen [51]. Furthermore these plants showed a more pronounced and earlier drop in (Glu+Asp)/(Gln+Asn) ratio during the progression of senescence indicating an additional adaption to low nitrogen conditions through enhanced nitrogen remobilization. In this experiment, also a significant increase in the ratio of hexose to sucrose was observed at the beginning of senescence which was higher in N-starved plants. This indicates that sugar-related senescence induction is dependent on the availability of nitrogen [51]. However, high sugar contents repress photosynthesis and can induce early SAG expression while late SAG expression is repressed. Diaz et al. (2005) [52] showed sugar accumulation to be lower in some recombinant inbred lines which display early leaf yellowing, thus pointing out a mayor function for sugar accumulation alone but the regulating function of the C/N balance during induction of monocarpic senescence is widely discussed. Recently, trehalose-6-phosphate (T6P) was identified as a main signaling component in this pathway. T6P inhibits the activity of Snf1-related protein kinase (SnRK1). Zhang et al. (2009) [53] showed the T6P/SnRK1 interaction in Arabidopsis seedling extracts and other young tissues treated with T6P. Additionally, Delatte et al. (2011) [54] confirmed the inhibition of SnRK1 by T6P with plants overexpressing the SnRK1 catalytic subunit gene *KIN10*. These plants were insensitive to trehalose treatments. Further verification of T6P as signaling molecule was provided by several studies. In wheat the interaction of T6P and SnRK1 has been suggested to play a role during grain filling [55]. Wingler et al. (2012) [56] conducted a study with *otsA* and *otsB* expressing Arabidopsis plants *otsA* encodes the bacterial T6P synthase gene, *otsB* the T6P phosphatase gene; therefore, overexpression leads to increasing or decreasing T6P contents, respectively. A significantly higher accumulation of glucose, fructose and sucrose was observed in *otsB* expressing plants and these plants displayed a delayed senescence phenotype. But most interestingly, these plants were rendered less susceptible to the induction of senescence-associated genes by sugar feeding in combination with low nitrogen supply, whereas *otsA* plants induced senescence and anthocyanin synthesis upon external supply of 2% glucose.

Another signaling component involved in senescence induction is light quantity and quality. Senescence can be induced by the darkening of individual leaves. However, darkening of the whole plant resulted in delay rather than in induction of leaf senescence in Arabidopsis and sunflower plants [57, 58]. Brouwer et al. (2012) [59] recently revealed the involvement of photoreceptors in dark and shading induced leaf responses. They applied different shading conditions to single leaves of Arabidopsis plants. Depending on the amount of light perceived, different biological programs were induced, leading to either acclimation to the new light conditions or leaf senescence. Furthermore, *phytochrome A* mutant lines displayed accelerated chlorophyll degradation under all shading conditions except darkness, displaying its involvement in the perception of and adaption to changing light conditions [59].

A tight linkage between stress response and leaf senescence is demonstrated by the function of several members of the NAC- and WRKY-family [60]. For example, *At NTL9 (NAC TRANSCRIPTION FACTOR LIKE 9)* mediates osmotic stress signaling during leaf senescence [61] and *At VNI2 (ANAC083)* has been shown to integrate abscisic acid (ABA)-mediated abiotic stress signals into leaf senescence [62].

Besides various other cues like the stage of plant development, pathogens, extreme temperatures, source-sink transitions and drought, the action of reactive oxygen species (ROS) has been shown to have a severe impact on the induction of leaf senescence. Cellular H_2O_2 levels increase at the onset of senescence due to a complex regulation of hydrogen peroxide scavenging enzymes [63]. The increase in intracellular H_2O_2 levels is initiated via the down-regulation of the expression of the hydrogen peroxide scavenging enzyme CATALASE2 by the transcription factor GBF1 (G-Box binding factor 1). In *gbf1* knock-out plants, the senescence specific elevation in H_2O_2 levels is absent leading to a significant delay of leaf senescence [64]. We have demonstrated recently using a specific *in vivo* hydrogen peroxide monitoring and scavenging system that the pivotal role of H_2O_2 during the induction of developmental leaf senescence in Arabidopsis is depending on the subcellular localization and concentration. Furthermore, a similar senescence-specific up-regulation of H_2O_2 levels and down-regulation of the respective scavenging enzymes was also observed in *Brassica napus* [65]. Knock-out and overexpression plants of *AtOSR1* (*ANAC059* or *ATNAC3*) or *AtJUB1* (*ANAC042*), which are both highly inducible by H_2O_2, were delayed or accelerated, respectively, concerning the onset of leaf senescence in which JUB1 also modulates cellular H_2O_2 levels [66, 67]. Besides their important role in disease resistance [68], several WRKY transcription factors have been suggested to have a striking role in the regulation of leaf senescence. For example AtWRKY53, a H_2O_2-responsive transcription factor, has been indicated to have a function as important control element during the onset of leaf senescence [69].

Conclusively, leaf senescence is governed not only by developmental age but a wide range of various different external and internal factors, biotic and abiotic influences, molecules and cues, which have to be integrated. Despite its enormous agricultural importance, our knowledge of these integrative mechanisms is still limited and needs much more efforts to get complete insight into the regulatory network controlling the onset and progression of leaf senescence.

3.1.1. N-uptake during senescence

Nitrogen uptake and partitioning after beginning anthesis varies greatly between different species and even between ecotypes. An analysis of different Arabidopsis accessions revealed that the fate of nitrogen absorbed during flowering can be different, depending on general N availability and accession. At low nitrogen concentrations most of the N assimilated post-flowering was allocated to the seeds, while under high N regimes the main part of it was distributed to the rosette leaves and successively lost in the dry remains, except for four tested accessions. N13, Sakata, Bl-1 and Oy-0 allocated the nitrogen taken up post-flowering also to the seeds under high N supply [70]. In wheat, a minor portion of grain N is derived from N uptake post-flowering, whereas up to 90-95% is remobilized from other plant tissues [3, 71]. In oilseed rape (*Brassica napus*) the induction of the reproductive phase is accompanied with a drastic down-regulation of nitrogen uptake systems. HATs and HATs + LATs activities are decreased thus almost resulting in an arrest of nitrogen uptake during seed filling and flowering [14, 72-74]. Grown under non-limiting nitrogen conditions, Arabidopsis displays a lowered nitrate influx during the reproductive stage in comparison to the influx during the vegetative stage [14]. Although many plants seem to continue N uptake during seed filling, this nitrogen is not always allocated to the seeds, thus rendering nitrogen remobilization from senescing organs a central component for the proper development of reproductive organs.

3.2. Nitrogen mobilization

3.2.1. *Senescence associated proteases*

Protein degradation is most likely the most important degradation process that occurs during senescence [75]. With a combined ^{15}N tracing/proteomics approach, Desclos et al. (2009) [76] have shown that HSP70, chaperonin10 and disulfide isomerase are synthesized during the whole progression of senescence in *B. napus* illustrating the necessity to prevent the aggregation of denatured proteins. In addition, almost all protease families have been associated with some aspects of plant senescence [75].

The aminopeptidase LAP2 has been characterized as exopeptidase liberating N-terminal leucine, methionine and phenylalanine. Arabidopsis *lap2* mutants displayed a significant change in amino acid contents. In particular, nitrogen rich AAs like glutamate and glutamine were dramatically reduced while leucine levels were the same as in wild type plants. Furthermore, a premature leaf senescence phenotype was observed in these plants. Different recombinant inbred lines, which are also modified in Glu, Gln, Asp and Asn contents, also show a senescence phenotype tempting the authors to speculate that the senescence phenotype of *lab2* might be related to a decreased turnover of defective proteins and the marked decrease of nitrogen rich AAs [77].

Chloroplast targeted proteases comprise proteases of the Lon, PreP, Clp, FtsH and DegP type [78-80]. Their substrates include, besides others, chlorophyll apoproteins like LHCII, the D1 protein of the photosystem II reaction center and Rubisco. The Clp protease complex is the most abundant stromal protease, where PreP is also located [78, 79]. Several catalytic subunits of the Clp proteases display up-regulated expression during dark-induced senescence in Arabidopsis, like e.g. ClpD/ERD1 and ClpC1. They possess sequence similarity to the chaperon HSP100 indicating that they might function as recognition subunit in the Clp protease complex to recruit denatured proteins [80]. FtsH proteases are thylakoid bound facing the stroma while Deg proteases are also thylakoid bound but facing stroma as well as thylakoid lumen [81, 82]. DegP2 is responsible for an initial cleavage of the D1 protein, where after FtsH proteases complete the full degradation [80, 83]. These two proteases belong to the family of serine proteases. In wheat, serine proteases are the most important family of proteases participating in N remobilization [84]. Subtilases have been reported to be highly expressed in barley during natural and senescence induced via artificial carbohydrate accumulation. Additionally induced proteases were SAG12, CND41-like, papain-like, serine carboxypeptidase III precursor, aspartic endopeptidases and others [85]. Roberts et al. (2012) [75] suggest a classification of senescence-associated proteases according to their expression profile and probable function during natural senescence. Class I includes all proteases being expressed in non-senescent and in senescent tissue. Although no senescence specific expression change can be observed, their continued expression in a catabolic environment displays their significance for a normal progression of senescence. Class II contains proteases being expressed at a low level in non-senescent tissue and induced upon senescence onset. Class III comprises proteases which are induced exclusively during senescence. This suggests a role in the late stages of senescence and a probable function in cell death execution. Class IV proteases constitute proteases transiently expressed during onset of senescence which could be involved in early breakdown processes like e.g. chloroplast dismantling. Finally, class V proteases are down-regulated during senescence. These enzymes are likely to fulfill housekeeping protein turnover and other proteolytic functions, which are no longer needed during the progression of leaf senescence [75].

3.2.2. Chloroplast dismantling

Chloroplasts are the first organelles to show visible symptoms of degradation processes during senescence. Containing up to 75% of total leaf nitrogen, chloroplasts are the main source for its remobilization [86]. Four different pathways have been proposed for chloroplast and chloroplastic protein degradation: I) endogenous proteases degrade proteins intra-plastidial, II) degradation of stroma fragments in an extraplastidic, non-autophagic pathway, as well as III) extraplastidic degradation by autophagy-associated pathways, and IV) autophagic degradation of entire plastids [87]. Chloroplast breakdown is not a chaotic decay, but rather an organized and selective process. As chloroplasts are one of the plants main ROS-producing organelles, and due to the potential phototoxicity of many chloroplastic components and their degradation intermediates, a coordinated dismantling process is necessary to prevent severe cell damage [88, 89].

Within these organelles Rubisco represents the most abundant protein. Its abundance exceeds the requirements for photosynthesis by far, thus a nitrogen storage function has been suggested for it [90]. In chloroplasts isolated from senescing leaves a 44 kDa fragment of Rubisco's large subunit accumulates, but seems not to be degraded further [91]. The chloroplastic aspartate protease CND41 has been shown to degrade denatured Rubisco, but not active Rubisco *in vitro* [92]. This protease might be involved directly in Rubisco degradation, as accumulation of CND41 correlates with loss of Rubisco [93]. However, tobacco CND41 antisense lines also show a dwarf phenotype, reduced gibberellin levels and reduced leaf expansion, thus this correlation could be an indirect effect through gibberellin homeostasis [94]. Rubisco containing bodies (RCB) have been found to be shuttling from the chloroplast to the central vacuole via an autophagy-dependent pathway [95]. The autophagy-dependency of these bodies was shown using *atg4a4b-1*mutants which are impaired in autophagy. Chloroplast fate was investigated in individually darkened leaves (IDLs) of wild type plants and *atg4a4b-1* mutants since individual darkening of leaves has been shown to rapidly induce senescence [57]. Wild type plants showed a decrease in chloroplast number and size as well as formation of RCBs. A*tg4a4b-1* mutant lines also displayed a decrease in chloroplast size but RCB formation was abolished and also the count of chloroplasts stayed constant.

However, Rubisco, nitrogen, soluble protein and chlorophyll contents decreased at almost the same rate in wild type plants as in *atg4a4b-1* mutant plants. This suggests alternative, autophagy-independent protein degradation pathways [96]. Lastly, despite the earlier mentioned 44 kDa Rubisco fragment observed in isolated chloroplasts, oxidative stress conditions might also initiate degradation of Rubisco's large subunit, as under these conditions the large subunit is split into a 37 and a 16 kDa fragment [97].

Besides the RCBs, senescence-associated vacuoles (SAVs) have been described. These vacuoles, enclosed by a single membrane layer, are enriched in Rubisco and display a high proteolytic activity at a pH more acidic than the central vacuole´s. SAVs are structurally not related to RCBs which posses a double layer membrane [95, 98]. The double layer membrane enclosing the RCBs appears to be derived from the chloroplast envelope [95]. Furthermore, SAV development seems to be autophagy-independent, as Arabidopsis *atapg7-1* mutant lines show normal SAV formation [98]. SAVs are only formed in leaf mesophyll cells. They are approximately 700 nm in diameter and can be labeled with antibodies against the (H+)-pyrophosphatase, an Arabidopsis vacuolar marker indicating these organelles indeed to be vacuoles [98]. Accumulation of stromal proteins in the SAVs was proven via plastid localized GFP which localized in SAVs in senescing tobacco leaves. In addition, high levels of chloroplastic glutamine synthase could be detected within these vacuoles [89]. Although the chlorophyll degradation pathway has been elucidated to a large extend and the first steps are regarded to occur within the plastid [88, 99], chlorophyll *a* has been found in SAVs under certain conditions, thus an alternative degradation pathway can be proposed [89]. Despite SAG12 has been shown to localize in SAVs, *sag12* mutant lines did neither show impairment in SAV formation nor in the proteolytic activity within the SAVs [98].

Even though chlorophyll represents about 2% of the total cellular nitrogen content [86], N fixed in chlorophyll is not exported from the leaf but rather remains in the vacuole [100]. However, around 20% N are fixed in proteins associated with or directly binding chlorophyll [88] and removal of chlorophyll seems to be a prerequisite for degradation of the corresponding apoproteins [88]. Pheophorbide a oxygenase (PAO) is an iron-dependent monooxygenase localized to the inner envelope of maturing gerontoplasts and catalyzes the conversion of pheophorbide a to red chlorophyll catabolites, one of the first steps during chlorophyll degradation. It represents a key control point in regulation of chlorophyll degradation [88, 101, 102]. In *pao* mutants and other stay green mutants affected in PAO activity and thus impaired chlorophyll degradation, this retention is accompanied with the accumulation of chlorophyll apoproteins like LHCII (see [88] and references within).

3.2.3. Autophagy

Autophagy plays a crucial role for nitrogen remobilization. The most striking phenotype of all *atg* mutants is hypersensitivity to nitrogen starvation ([103] and references within). Furthermore, an age dependent early senescence phenotype can be observed. As autophagy is involved in molecule degradation one would expect delayed senescence if this pathway is blocked. One hypothesis explaining this contradiction is that the autophagy pathway is normally activated at an early stage of senescence starting to degrade plastid proteins while leaving the photosynthetic apparatus intact. However, when autophagy is blocked, it is speculated that autophagy-independent pathways for chloroplast protein degradation might be activated untimely leading to premature chloroplast and chlorophyll degradation and thus to an early senescence phenotype [104]. Recently, Guiboileau et al. (2012) [103] conducted a study on the impact of *atg* mutants (*atg5, atg9* and RNAi18) on nitrogen remobilization. These plants were grown under ample and low nitrate conditions. In comparison to wild type plants the dry weight as well as the seed weight was lowered. However, when calculating the harvest index, *atg* mutants did not display a significant difference, except for the *atg5* mutant line at low N conditions. When the nitrogen use and remobilization efficiency was investigated via ^{15}N tracing experiments, all *atg* lines showed a decrease in this feature. It was demonstrated that remobilization was significantly impaired, as N contents in the plants dry remains were enriched and ^{15}N previously partitioned to the leaves was not mobilized to the seeds. To verify that this impairment rests on an autophagy defect and not on premature senescence and cell death symptoms, *atg5* mutants were combined with two SA signaling mutants, *sid2* and *nahG,* overriding the early senescence phenotype. These mutants reached nearly wild type biomass levels, but did not compensate the decrease in NRE. These results and the finding that autophagy regulates SA levels in a negative feedback loop [105] suggest, that the premature senescence phenotype in *atg* mutants is at least in part mediated by increased SA levels [104]. Conclusively, blocked autophagy pathways might result in an early senescence phenotype because of the accumulation of damaged and thus potentially toxic molecules in combination with a missing negative feedback on SA levels leading to cell death and activation of alternative pathways for bulk protein degradation.

3.2.4. Re-assimilation and translocation of salvaged nitrogen

As mentioned above, chloroplastic glutamine synthetase (GS2), GOGAT, NiR and Rubisco are targeted for rapid degradation already during early phases of senescence, disrupting primary nitrogen assimilation. Proteolysis in the vacuole feeds into the cellular pool of free AAs during the progression of senescence. The steady-state concentrations of free AAs depend on the rate of their release due to proteolysis and their efflux into growing structures [106]. Soudry et al. (2005) [106] have utilized a bioluminescence assay combined with auxotrophic bacteria for the detection of free tryptophan levels. They assumed that tryptophan reflects the overall pool of free AAs, as it is not modified before its export into sink organs. An accumulation of free AAs was observed in detached oat and Arabidopsis leaves. While attached oat leaves showed a gradual decrease in tryptophan levels during further progression of senescence, the attached Arabidopsis leaves did not or only due to membrane leakage resulting from the experimental procedure. The authors concluded that not only source strength but also sink strength is important for successful nutrient remobilization and suggested that the small reproductive organs of Arabidopsis exerted too weak sink strength. However, these findings might be related to the experimental design, as Arabidopsis does indeed remobilize N for seed filling [70] and Diaz et al. (2005) [52] reported decreasing levels for several AAs during the progression of leaf senescence in Arabidopsis. Protein breakdown increases free AAs in the cell. While some seem to be exported without prior modification, many are probably modified, hydrolyzed or interconverted. Expressional profiling revealed that, besides others, the cytosolic GS1, glutamate dehydrogenase (GDH) and asparagine synthetase (AS) are specifically induced during senescence [14]. A series of transamination reactions would result in an accumulation of glutamate, which could serve as substrate for GDH. Deamination of glutamate via GDH provides then 2OG and ammonia. NH_3 could then in turn be used as substrate for cytosolic GS1, giving rise to glutamine, which is one of the major nitrogen transport forms during nutrient remobilization. In fact many studies strengthen a positive correlation between GS activity and yield as well as grain and stem N content. Martin et al. (2006) [107] identified two cytosolic glutamine synthetase isoforms in maize which have a major impact on kernel size and yield. In wheat, GS activity was also positively linked with grain and stem N content [71]. Recently, two rice varieties with different levels of GS2 activity were analyzed and plants with higher activity displayed less NH_3 emission due to photorespiration and a better ability to recycle and reassimilate ammonia within the plant [108]. In barley amino acid permeases (AAP) seem to play a significant role during N retranslocation and grain filling. Recent RNA-Seq data revealed an overrepresentation of this gene family in both source and sink tissues. Furthermore, the grain-specific HvAAP3, which was also identified in this study, has high sequence similarity to Arabidopsis AAP1 and AAP8, which have been already shown to be involved in seed N supply (see [109] and references within).

Asparagine amounts also increase significantly in whole rosettes darkened for several days as well as in senescent leaves (see e.g. [1, 80]). Besides the senescence specific up-regulation of AS, pyruvate orthophosphate dikinase (PPDK) expression is also significantly increased during dark-induced senescence [80]. PPDK might have a role in carbon salvage after lipid degradation, thus Lin and Wu (2004) [80] also investigated other pathways possibly involved in this process. Remarkably, they found only a few components of these pathways to be up-regulated and many others even down-regulated. Based on their expressional profiling data, they postulated a alternative pathway for asparagine synthesis, where PPDK delivers metabolic precursors [80]. Additionally, seed protein contents were elevated and viability of seedlings was increased on nitrogen-limiting media in Arabidopsis *ASN1* overexpressor lines (*35S*::*ASN1*). Furthermore, they observed more Asn to be allocated to flowers and developing siliques and also higher Asn contents in phloem exudates [80, 110].

Nitrogen is not only remobilized from older leaves via amino acids. Nitrate and ammonia are also translocated to developing sink tissues. Fan et al. (2009) [111] identified a nitrate transporter (NRT1-7) which is involved in remobilization processes. Arabidopsis *nrt1-7* mutants displayed retarded growth under nitrogen starvation conditions. Also the spatial expression of this transporter in phloem tissue of older leaves and the expressional induction upon nitrogen starvation points out its function in nitrogen remobilization. Finally, the inability of *nrt1-7* mutants to remobilize ^{15}N from old to young leaves and the high accumulation of nitrate in old leaves in this mutants further underlines this assumption [111]. Another nitrate transporter involved in remobilization is NRT2-4. This transporter acts in the high-affinity range and its expression is also induced upon nitrogen starvation. Additionally, *nrt2-4* mutant lines had lower phloem sap nitrate contents. However, *nrt2-4* mutants were not altered in growth or development, indicating that the decreased NO_3-levels are not limiting for the adaption to N starvation and most likely functionally redundant transporter systems exist [40].

4. Reactive oxygen and nitrogen species in signaling

Reactive oxygen and nitrogen species (ROS, RNS) play a central role in many aspects of plant development and response to environmental influences. These include among others responses to wounding, pathogen infection, drought and water stress, high salinity, cold and heat. In the case of ROS, research has focused especially on H_2O_2. As this reactive oxygen molecule is relatively long lived (~1 ms half life), small and uncharged, and thus is able to pass membranes, a central position in various signaling pathways has been attributed to it. Nitric oxide (NO) has been shown to be involved in many of the H_2O_2-mediated pathways in either a synergistic or antagonistic mode of action. In the following we will briefly introduce the production and scavenging mechanisms for this two reactive oxygen and nitrogen compounds and their interplay in regulation of developmental processes, stress responses and senescence will be outlined.

4.1. ROS and RNS: Molecule types, production and scavenging

Many of the reactive oxygen species in the cell are formed as toxic byproducts of metabolic processes. Photorespiration and β-oxidation of fatty acids produce H_2O_2 in peroxisomes and glyoxisomes, which is normally scavenged by an extensive protection system mainly consisting of catalases (CAT) and ascorbate peroxidases (APX). Xanthine oxidase generates superoxide anions in the peroxisomes, which is converted by superoxide dismutases (SOD) into O_2 and H_2O_2. Chloroplasts are the main site for ROS production in plants. Due to the photooxidative nature of many of their components they can give rise to superoxide radicals, hydrogen peroxide, hydroxyl radicals and singlet oxygen. ROS produced in the chloroplasts are mainly scavenged by the ascorbate-glutathione cycle [112]. SODs scavenge superoxide anions and dismutate them to O_2 and H_2O_2, which is then in turn reduced to water by the action of ascorbate peroxidase and ascorbate. The resulting monodehydro-ascorbate (MDHA) is regenerated either via the MDHA reductase (MDHAR) under the use of NADPH or it spontaneously converts into dehydroascorbate (DHA) which is then reduced to ascorbate again via the DHA reductase (DHAR). DHAR uses glutathione (GSH) as second substrate. The reduced state of GSH is reconstituted by glutathione reductase (GR). Excess oxidized GSSG seems to be exported from the cytosol to the central vacuole and the chloroplasts to maintain a reduced environment and redox homeostasis in the cytosol and possibly the nucleus [113]. Finally, superoxide radicals can be produced as a byproduct during respiration in mitochondria. Here, also SOD and the ascorbate-glutathione cycle removes the ROS. Further ROS scavenging in this organelle is mediated by peroxiredoxins and thioredoxins, as it is also observed in chloroplasts. Additionally, non-enzymatic components like tocopherols, flavonoids, ascorbic acid and others are employed in the extensive and elaborate ROS detoxification system (reviewed in [114-119]). Under optimal growth conditions,

ROS production is relatively low; however, during stress, the production of ROS is rapidly enhanced [120].

Active production of ROS or the so called "oxidative burst" is initiated upon several stresses and developmental stimuli. The main enzymes generating these ROS are the respiratory burst oxidase homologs (RBOH) [121]. In a NADPH-dependent reaction they form O_2^- in the apoplast. This is then converted by SODs to H_2O_2. The function of the 10 different RBOH proteins identified in Arabidopsis [122] is important in various developmental and regulatory processes. Root elongation is reduced in *atrbohD/F* mutants [122]. ROS produced upon pathogen attack are generated by RBOHs (see for example [123]). Also the response to heavy metals seems to be at least in part mediated by RBOH proteins. Cadmium treated sunflower leaf discs showed an altered expression and activity of the NADPH oxidase [124]. The function of these proteins is often associated with the action of Ca^{2+}. Arabidopsis *rbohC/rhd2* mutants displayed lowered ROS contents in growing root hairs and a distortion in Ca^{2+} uptake due to a missing activation of Ca^{2+} channels [125], although for the rice RBOHB homolog calcium was needed to activate the oxidase itself [126].

Reactive nitrogen species (RNS) comprise NO and NO-derived molecules as di-nitrogen trioxide, nitrogen dioxide, peroxynitrite, S-nitrosothiols and others [127]. NO production in plant cells is under continuous debate. Especially the existence of a plant nitric oxide synthase (NOS) is a controversial topic. Until today, there is no clear proof for the existence of NOS in plants although there is indirect evidence through the application of NOS inhibitors, which have been established for mammalian cells (e.g. L-NAME a L-arginine analogue) in combination with NR inhibitors, or the measurement of NOS-like activity, like the conversion of L-arginine to citrulline, where NO is assumed to be produced at the same time [128-130]. AtNOS1 was identified in 2003 by Guo et al. (2003) [131], but is under controversial discussion ever since. Indeed, *atnos1* mutant plants do exhibit significantly lower NO contents, a chlorotic phenotype in seedlings which can be rescued by NO application and an early-senescence phenotype, but expression of the corresponding genes from Arabidopsis, maize and rice revealed no NOS activity *in-vitro*, and even the mammalian orthologous displayed no NOS function [132]. Thus *AtNOS1* was renamed to *AtNOA1* (NO associated 1). Nevertheless, there are other enzymatic ways known to produce NO. NR was found to be able to generate NO. It was shown to be involved in NO generation during the transition to flowering Arabidopsis *nr1* and *nr2* mutants display a low endogenous NO content [133, 134]. Additionally, a NR- and NiR-independent pathway of NO production has been proposed via electron carriers of the mitochondrial respiratory chain [135] and an oxidation-associated pathway for NO synthesis has been suggested as hydroxylamines can be oxidized by superoxide and H_2O_2 generating NO [136].

Despite all the controversy on the topic of NO generation, it seems clear, that there are many ways to generate NO in plant cells and the pivotal role in many regulatory pathways cannot be denied. Involvement in fruit ripening, leaf senescence, flowering and stomatal closure and many other processes has been shown ([129] and references within).

4.2. ROS and RNS: Signaling

The role of H_2O_2 and NO during the onset of leaf senescence has been investigated in many studies. Recently, an upstream regulator of the ROS network during ABA-mediated drought-induced leaf senescence has been identified. The drought-responsive NAC transcription factor AtNTL4 (ANAC053) has been shown to promote ROS production by directly binding to promoters of genes encoding ROS biosynthetic enzymes [137]. In guard cells, an ABA-H_2O_2-NO signaling cascade has been proposed for stomatal closure. H_2O_2-induced generation of NO in guard cells has been reported for mung bean [138], Arabidopsis [139] and other plant species (see for example [140]). Removal of H_2O_2 as well as the blocking of calcium channels was able to suppress NO generation [138, 141]. A further interaction of NO and H_2O_2 was studied in tomato (*Lycopersicon esculentum* Mill. cv. "Perkoz") where the effect of application of exogenous NO scavengers and generators was analyzed in combination with *Botrytis cinerea* inoculation. NO generators specifically reduced H_2O_2 generation and thus allowed the infection to spread significantly under control conditions and in comparison to NO scavenger pre-treated leaves [142]. Moreover, cytoplasmic H_2O_2 can also directly activate a specific Arabidopsis MAP triple kinase, AtANP1, which initiates a phosphorylation cascade involving two stress AtMAPKs, AtMPK3 and AtMPK6 [143]. A direct interaction between AtMPK6 and AtNR2 during lateral root development has been shown *in-vitro* and *in-vivo*. During this interaction MPK6 phosphorylates and thus activates NR2 resulting in enhanced NO production [144]. Finally, another point of crosstalk between the NO and H_2O_2 signaling pathways has been referred to by positional cloning of the rice *NOE1*. This gene codes for a rice catalase, a knock-out leads to increased H_2O_2 contents which in turn enhance the activity of NR, resulting in elevated NO concentrations. The removal of excess NO ameliorated the cell death symptoms of the *noe1* mutants pointing out a cooperative function of H_2O_2 and NO during induction of PCD. Here, specifically S-nitrosylated proteins were identified, and overexpression of a rice S-nitrosoglutathione reductase could also alleviate the cell death symptoms [145].

Senescence-inhibiting features of NO have long been recognized, while H_2O_2 has often been attributed with senescence-promoting features. Exogenous NO application extends postharvest life of fruits and vegetables and, during leaf maturation in pea, NO contents gradually decrease [146, 147]. Furthermore, NO-deficient mutants display an early-senescence phenotype and the heterologues expression of an NO-degrading enzyme in Arabidopsis also leads to early leaf senescence and SAG up-regulation, which could be inhibited by external supply of NO [148]. Remarkably, the senescence delaying features of NO might be achieved due its ability to scavenge various kinds of ROS. In barley aleuron cells, NO has been shown to act as an antioxidant and thus alleviating GA-mediated PCD induction [149].

4.3. Specificity in ROS and RNS signaling

Some amino acids are more susceptible for modification by ROS and RNS than others. For example cysteins are often found to be preferentially oxidized. These residues are sensitive for ROS-derived protein carbonylation and RNS-mediated nitrosylation (-SNO) and glutahionylation. Additionally, sulfenic acid and disulfide formation also can be mediated via ROS and RNS on these residues. Tryptophane residues have been shown to be specifically di-oxygenized in plant mitochondria, thus forming N-formylkynurenine. The proteins found to be specifically oxygenized did, with one exception, all posses redox-activity or were involved in redox-active proteins [150]. Another good example for this specificity is Rubisco. Preferential oxidation of certain cysteine residues mediates the binding of Rubisco to the chloroplast envelope, thus causing catalytic inactivation and marking it for degradation [151, 152]. Recently, it has been shown, that chloroplast peroxidases are present in an inactivated form and become activated in part by proteolytic cleavage upon a H_2O_2 signal; in combination with newly synthesized peroxidases, they regulate plastidial ROS content in neem (*Azadirachta indica* A. juss) chloroplasts [153]. This displays a specificity of ROS induced processes, rather than undirected, detrimental impacts. However, how the cell responds differentially to the variety of H_2O_2 signals in different signaling pathways is still unclear. With regard to leaf senescence induction, a dependency of H_2O_2-mediated effects on the subcellular location was discovered. By using an *in-vivo* H_2O_2-scavenging system, we manipulated H_2O_2 contents in the cytosol and peroxisomes in Arabidopsis. While both lines showed lowered H_2O_2 contents and a delayed leaf senescence phenotype, the delay of the cytoplasmic line was more pronounced, despite the higher expression of the peroxisomal transgene [65]. Furthermore, lowering mitochondrial H_2O_2 production by blocking cytochrome *c* dependent respiration with the fungal toxin antimycin A had no effect on induction of leaf senescence [154]. Since senescence is predominantly regulated on transcriptional level, the cytoplasmic compartment might have a direct influence on redox regulation of transcription factors. Expression of the MAP triple kinase1 (*MEKK1*) of Arabidopsis can also be induced by H_2O_2 and shows its expression maximum during onset of leaf senescence [155]. Whether H_2O_2 induced expression of SAGs is transduced by MAPK signaling or directly by redox-sensitive transcription factors has yet to be elucidated.

Moreover, the already mentioned evidence of numerous selective oxidation reactions on specific amino acid residues depending on the type of ROS/RNS might lead to the degradation of the damaged proteins, thus generating distinct peptide patterns. These peptides would contain information being ROS- and source-specific (see [150] and references within). Spatial control might also be a source of specificity, as for example RBOH proteins are membrane bound and, therefore, localization of the ROS signal could be highly specific. Additionally, through the extensive detoxification system, ROS signals also might be spatially confined. In contrast, ROS signal auto-propagation over long distances via RBOHD induced by various stimuli has been shown in Arabidopsis [156]. Interestingly, temporal oscillation of ROS bursts has been observed to modulate root tip growth of Arabidopsis root hairs [157]. Finally, integration of metabolic reactions also seems to be a convenient way of specific signaling. Local blockage or enhancement of certain pathways would lead to the accumulation of intermediates, which in turn could serve for signaling functions (reviewed in [158]).

5. Concluding remarks

The intriguing connection between efficient nutrient remobilization and progression of leaf senescence is obvious. The correct timing of onset and progression of senescence has great influence on seed and fruit development and viability. Therefore, manipulating leaf senescence seems to be a promising trait to increase yield in various crop species. Functional stay green traits can prolong carbon assimilation and thus increase yield. However, a too strong delay in leaf senescence might hamper nutrient and especially nitrogen remobilization from the leaves. For various wheat mutants, Derkx et al. (2012) [159] speculated that the stay green phenotype might be associated with a decrease in grain N sink strength. Gpc-B1, a QTL locus in wheat, which is among others associated with increased grain protein content, has been shown to encode a NAC transcription factor (*NAM-B1*). It accelerates senescence and enhances nutrient remobilization from leaves. RNA interference mediated silencing of multiple homologues resulted in a delay of leaf senescence by approximately 3 weeks and decreased grain protein, iron and zinc content by more than 30% [160]. This indicates that the relation between senescence and nitrogen mobilization is very complicated and cannot be modified as easy as expected.

Besides QTL selection, transgenic approaches to increase nitrogen use efficiency in crop plants have been extensively studied. For example expression of alanine aminotransferase and asparagine synthase often resulted in enhanced seed protein content and higher seed yield. Increased cytokinin biosynthesis almost always resulted in delayed senescence and was sometimes associated with higher seed yield, seed protein content and increased biomass. Expression of amino acid permease from *Vicia faba* under the *LeB4* promoter increased the seed size by 20-30%, as well as the abundance of nitrogen rich AAs and the content of seed storage proteins in the seeds (reviewed in [161]).

Nevertheless, although transgenic approaches have proven to enhance nitrogen use efficiencies and yield quantity as well as quality, these techniques have to cope with general skepticism on the consumer's side. Although approval for the agricultural use of genetically modified organisms has been extensively performed like e.g. in the Swiss National Research program NRP 59 (Benefits and risks of the deliberated release of genetically modified plants) clearly indicating a low risk and a enormously high potential of transgenic crop plants, problems with the acceptance of this technology, especially in Europe, still have to be faced.

Author details

Stefan Bieker and Ulrike Zentgraf

General Genetics, University of Tuebingen, Tuebingen, Germany

References

[1] Diaz C, Lemaître T, Christ A, Azzopardi M, Kato Y, Sato F, et al. Nitrogen Recycling and Remobilization Are Differentially Controlled by Leaf Senescence and Development Stage in Arabidopsis under Low Nitrogen Nutrition. Plant Physiology. 2008 July 2008;147(3):1437-49.

[2] Luquez VMC, Sasal Y, Medrano M, Martín MI, Mujica M, Guiamét JJ. Quantitative trait loci analysis of leaf and plant longevity in Arabidopsis thaliana. Journal of Experimental Botany. 2006 March 2006;57(6):1363-72.

[3] Kichey T, Hirel B, Heumez E, Dubois F, Le Gouis J. In winter wheat (Triticum aestivum L.), post-anthesis nitrogen uptake and remobilisation to the grain correlates with agronomic traits and nitrogen physiological markers. Field Crop Res. 2007 Apr 30;102(1):22-32.

[4] Breeze E, Harrison E, McHattie S, Hughes L, Hickman R, Hill C, et al. High-resolution temporal profiling of transcripts during Arabidopsis leaf senescence reveals a distinct chronology of processes and regulation. Plant Cell. 2011 Mar;23(3):873-94.

[5] Lim PO, Kim HJ, Nam HG. Leaf senescence. Annual Review of Plant Biology. 2007;58:115-36.

[6] Grbic V, Bleecker AB. Ethylene Regulates the Timing of Leaf Senescence in Arabidopsis. Plant Journal. 1995 Oct;8(4):595-602.

[7] Kim HJ, Ryu H, Hong SH, Woo HR, Lim PO, Lee IC, et al. Cytokinin-mediated control of leaf longevity by AHK3 through phosphorylation of ARR2 in Arabidopsis. P Natl Acad Sci USA. 2006 Jan 17;103(3):814-9.

[8] Lee IC, Hong SW, Whang SS, Lim PO, Nam HG, Koo JC. Age-Dependent Action of an ABA-Inducible Receptor Kinase, RPK1, as a Positive Regulator of Senescence in Arabidopsis Leaves. Plant and Cell Physiology. 2011 Apr;52(4):651-62.

[9] Osakabe Y, Maruyama K, Seki M, Satou M, Shinozaki K, Yamaguchi-Shinozaki K. Leucine-rich repeat receptor-like kinase1 is a key membrane-bound regulator of abscisic acid early signaling in Arabidopsis. Plant Cell. 2005 Apr;17(4):1105-19.

[10] Osakabe Y, Mizuno S, Tanaka H, Maruyama K, Osakabe K, Todaka D, et al. Overproduction of the Membrane-bound Receptor-like Protein Kinase 1, RPK1, Enhances Abiotic Stress Tolerance in Arabidopsis. J Biol Chem. 2010 Mar 19;285(12):9190-201.

[11] Division DoEaSAP. World Population Prospects: The 2008 Revision, Highlights. Popul Dev Rev. 2010 Dec;36(4):854-5.

[12] Tilman D, Cassman KG, Matson PA, Naylor R, Polasky S. Agricultural sustainability and intensive production practices. Nature. 2002 Aug 8;418(6898):671-7.

[13] Ribaudo M, Delgado J, Hansen LT, Livingston M, Mosheim R, Williamson JM. Nitrogen in Agricultural Systems: Implications for Conservation Policy. United States Department of Agriculture, Economic Research Service, 2011.

[14] Masclaux-Daubresse C, Daniel-Vedele F, Dechorgnat J, Chardon F, Gaufichon L, Suzuki A. Nitrogen uptake, assimilation and remobilization in plants: challenges for sustainable and productive agriculture. Ann Bot. 2010 Jun;105(7):1141-57.

[15] Good AG, Shrawat AK, Muench DG. Can less yield more? Is reducing nutrient input into the environment compatible with maintaining crop production? Trends in Plant Science. 2004 Dec;9(12):597-605.

[16] Peoples MB, Freney JR, Mosier AR. Minimizing gaseous losses of nitrogen. In: Bacon PE, editor. Nitrogen fertilization in the environment. New York et al.: Marcel Dekker, Inc.; 1995. p. 565-602.

[17] Bogard M, Jourdan M, Allard V, Martre P, Perretant MR, Ravel C, et al. Anthesis date mainly explained correlations between post-anthesis leaf senescence, grain yield, and grain protein concentration in a winter wheat population segregating for flowering time QTLs. Journal of Experimental Botany. 2011 Jun;62(10):3621-36.

[18] Oury FX, Godin C. Yield and grain protein concentration in bread wheat: how to use the negative relationship between the two characters to identify favourable genotypes? Euphytica. 2007 Sep;157(1-2):45-57.

[19] Maathuis FJM. Physiological functions of mineral macronutrients. Current Opinion in Plant Biology. 2009 Jun;12(3):250-8.

[20] De Angeli A, Monachello D, Ephritikhine G, Frachisse JM, Thomine S, Gambale F, et al. The nitrate/proton antiporter AtCLCa mediates nitrate accumulation in plant vacuoles. Nature. 2006 Aug 24;442(7105):939-42.

[21] von der Fecht-Bartenbach J, Bogner M, Dynowski M, Ludewig U. CLC-b-Mediated NO3-/H+ Exchange Across the Tonoplast of Arabidopsis Vacuoles. Plant and Cell Physiology. 2010 Jun;51(6):960-8.

[22] Tsay YF, Chiu CC, Tsai CB, Ho CH, Hsu PK. Nitrate transporters and peptide transporters. Febs Letters. 2007 May 25;581(12):2290-300.

[23] Huang NC, Liu KH, Lo HJ, Tsay YF. Cloning and functional characterization of an Arabidopsis nitrate transporter gene that encodes a constitutive component of low-affinity uptake. Plant Cell. 1999 Aug;11(8):1381-92.

[24] Touraine B, Glass ADM. NO3- and ClO3- fluxes in the chl1-5 mutant of Arabidopsis thaliana - Does the CHL1-5 gene encode a low-affinity NO3- transporter? Plant Physiology. 1997 May;114(1):137-44.

[25] Tsay YF, Schroeder JI, Feldmann KA, Crawford NM. The Herbicide Sensitivity Gene Chl1 of Arabidopsis Encodes a Nitrate-Inducible Nitrate Transporter. Cell. 1993 Mar 12;72(5):705-13.

[26] Liu KH, Huang CY, Tsay YF. CHL1 is a dual-affinity nitrate transporter of arabidopsis involved in multiple phases of nitrate uptake. Plant Cell. 1999 May;11(5):865-74.

[27] Wang RC, Liu D, Crawford NM. The Arabidopsis CHL1 protein plays a major role in high-affinity nitrate uptake. P Natl Acad Sci USA. 1998 Dec 8;95(25):15134-9.

[28] Liu KH, Tsay YF. Switching between the two action modes of the dual-affinity nitrate transporter CHL1 by phosphorylation. EMBO J. 2003 Mar 3;22(5):1005-13.

[29] Ho CH, Lin SH, Hu HC, Tsay YF. CHL1 functions as a nitrate sensor in plants. Cell. 2009 Sep 18;138(6):1184-94.

[30] Lin SH, Kuo HF, Canivenc G, Lin CS, Lepetit M, Hsu PK, et al. Mutation of the Arabidopsis NRT1.5 nitrate transporter causes defective root-to-shoot nitrate transport. Plant Cell. 2008 Sep;20(9):2514-28.

[31] Chiu CC, Lin CS, Hsia AP, Su RC, Lin HL, Tsay YF. Mutation of a nitrate transporter, AtNRT1:4, results in a reduced petiole nitrate content and altered leaf development. Plant & cell physiology. 2004 Sep;45(9):1139-48.

[32] Almagro A, Lin SH, Tsay YF. Characterization of the Arabidopsis nitrate transporter NRT1.6 reveals a role of nitrate in early embryo development. Plant Cell. 2008 Dec; 20(12):3289-99.

[33] Li JY, Fu YL, Pike SM, Bao J, Tian W, Zhang Y, et al. The Arabidopsis nitrate transporter NRT1.8 functions in nitrate removal from the xylem sap and mediates cadmium tolerance. Plant Cell. 2010 May;22(5):1633-46.

[34] Wang YY, Tsay YF. Arabidopsis Nitrate Transporter NRT1.9 Is Important in Phloem Nitrate Transport. Plant Cell. 2011 May;23(5):1945-57.

[35] Filleur S, Dorbe MF, Cerezo M, Orsel M, Granier F, Gojon A, et al. An Arabidopsis T-DNA mutant affected in Nrt2 genes is impaired in nitrate uptake. Febs Letters. 2001 Feb 2;489(2-3):220-4.

[36] Little DY, Rao HY, Oliva S, Daniel-Vedele F, Krapp A, Malamy JE. The putative high-affinity nitrate transporter NRT2.1 represses lateral root initiation in response to nutritional cues. P Natl Acad Sci USA. 2005 Sep 20;102(38):13693-8.

[37] Zhou JJ, Fernandez E, Galvan A, Miller AJ. A high affinity nitrate transport system from Chlamydomonas requires two gene products. Febs Letters. 2000 Jan 28;466(2-3): 225-7.

[38] Orsel M, Chopin F, Leleu O, Smith SJ, Krapp A, Daniel-Vedele F, et al. Characterization of a two-component high-affinity nitrate uptake system in Arabidopsis. Physiology and protein-protein interaction. Plant Physiology. 2006 Nov;142(3):1304-17.

[39] Chopin F, Orsel M, Dorbe MF, Chardon F, Truong HN, Miller AJ, et al. The Arabidopsis ATNRT2.7 nitrate transporter controls nitrate content in seeds. Plant Cell. 2007 May;19(5):1590-602.

[40] Kiba T, Feria-Bourrellier AB, Lafouge F, Lezhneva L, Boutet-Mercey S, Orsel M, et al. The Arabidopsis nitrate transporter NRT2.4 plays a double role in roots and shoots of nitrogen-starved plants. Plant Cell. 2012 Jan;24(1):245-58.

[41] Loque D, von Wiren N. Regulatory levels for the transport of ammonium in plant roots. J Exp Bot. 2004 Jun;55(401):1293-305.

[42] Yuan L, Loque D, Ye F, Frommer WB, von Wiren N. Nitrogen-dependent posttranscriptional regulation of the ammonium transporter AtAMT1;1. Plant Physiol. 2007 Feb;143(2):732-44.

[43] Loque D, Yuan L, Kojima S, Gojon A, Wirth J, Gazzarrini S, et al. Additive contribution of AMT1;1 and AMT1;3 to high-affinity ammonium uptake across the plasma membrane of nitrogen-deficient Arabidopsis roots. Plant J. 2006 Nov;48(4):522-34.

[44] Kaiser BN, Rawat SR, Siddiqi MY, Masle J, Glass AD. Functional analysis of an Arabidopsis T-DNA "knockout" of the high-affinity NH4(+) transporter AtAMT1;1. Plant Physiol. 2002 Nov;130(3):1263-75.

[45] Okumoto S, Pilot G. Amino Acid Export in Plants: A Missing Link in Nitrogen Cycling. Molecular Plant. 2011 February 15, 2011.

[46] Schjoerring JK, Husted S, Mack G, Mattsson M. The regulation of ammonium translocation in plants. J Exp Bot. 2002 Apr;53(370):883-90.

[47] Zheng Z-L. Carbon and nitrogen nutrient balance signaling in plants. Plant Signaling & Behavior. 2009;4(7):584-91.

[48] Lawlor DW. Carbon and nitrogen assimilation in relation to yield: mechanisms are the key to understanding production systems. Journal of Experimental Botany. 2002 April 15, 2002;53(370):773-87.

[49] Dechorgnat J, Nguyen CT, Armengaud P, Jossier M, Diatloff E, Filleur S, et al. From the soil to the seeds: the long journey of nitrate in plants. J Exp Bot. 2011 Feb;62(4): 1349-59.

[50] Wingler A, Purdy S, MacLean JA, Pourtau N. The role of sugars in integrating environmental signals during the regulation of leaf senescence. J Exp Bot. 2006;57(2): 391-9.

[51] Aguera E, Cabello P, de la Haba P. Induction of leaf senescence by low nitrogen nutrition in sunflower (Helianthus annuus) plants. Physiol Plant. 2010 Mar;138(3): 256-67.

[52] Diaz C, Purdy S, Christ A, Morot-Gaudry J-F, Wingler A, Masclaux-Daubresse C. Characterization of Markers to Determine the Extent and Variability of Leaf Senescence in Arabidopsis. A Metabolic Profiling Approach. Plant Physiology. 2005 June 2005;138(2):898-908.

[53] Zhang Y, Primavesi LF, Jhurreea D, Andralojc PJ, Mitchell RAC, Powers SJ, et al. Inhibition of SNF1-Related Protein Kinase1 Activity and Regulation of Metabolic Pathways by Trehalose-6-Phosphate. Plant Physiology. 2009 April 2009;149(4):1860-71.

[54] Delatte TL, Sedijani P, Kondou Y, Matsui M, de Jong GJ, Somsen GW, et al. Growth Arrest by Trehalose-6-Phosphate: An Astonishing Case of Primary Metabolite Control over Growth by Way of the SnRK1 Signaling Pathway. Plant Physiology. 2011 September 1, 2011;157(1):160-74.

[55] Martinez-Barajas E, Delatte T, Schluepmann H, de Jong GJ, Somsen GW, Nunes C, et al. Wheat Grain Development Is Characterized by Remarkable Trehalose 6-Phosphate Accumulation Pregrain Filling: Tissue Distribution and Relationship to SNF1-Related Protein Kinase1 Activity. Plant Physiology. 2011 May;156(1):373-81.

[56] Wingler A, Delatte TL, O'Hara LE, Primavesi LF, Jhurreea D, Paul MJ, et al. Trehalose 6-Phosphate Is Required for the Onset of Leaf Senescence Associated with High Carbon Availability. Plant Physiology. 2012 Mar;158(3):1241-51.

[57] Weaver LM, Amasino RM. Senescence is induced in individually darkened Arabidopsis leaves but inhibited in whole darkened plants. Plant Physiology. 2001 Nov; 127(3):876-86.

[58] Ono K, Nishi Y, Watanabe A, Terashima I. Possible Mechanisms of Adaptive Leaf Senescence. Plant Biology. 2001;3(3):234-43.

[59] Brouwer B, Ziolkowska A, Bagard M, Keech O, Gardestrom P. The impact of light intensity on shade-induced leaf senescence. Plant Cell and Environment. 2012 Jun; 35(6):1084-98.

[60] Olsen AN, Ernst HA, Leggio LL, Skriver K. NAC transcription factors: structurally distinct, functionally diverse. Trends Plant Sci. 2005 Feb;10(2):79-87.

[61] Yoon HK, Kim SG, Kim SY, Park CM. Regulation of leaf senescence by NTL9-mediated osmotic stress signaling in Arabidopsis. Molecules and cells. 2008 May 31;25(3): 438-45.

[62] Yang SD, Seo PJ, Yoon HK, Park CM. The Arabidopsis NAC transcription factor VNI2 integrates abscisic acid signals into leaf senescence via the COR/RD genes. Plant Cell. 2011 Jun;23(6):2155-68.

[63] Zimmermann P, Heinlein C, Orendi G, Zentgraf U. Senescence-specific regulation of catalases in Arabidopsis thaliana (L.) Heynh. Plant Cell Environ. 2006 Jun;29(6): 1049-60.

[64] Smykowski A, Zimmermann P, Zentgraf U. G-Box binding factor1 reduces CATALASE2 expression and regulates the onset of leaf senescence in Arabidopsis. Plant Physiol. 2010 Jul;153(3):1321-31.

[65] Bieker S, Riester L, Stahl M, Franzaring J, Zentgraf U. Senescence-specific Alteration of Hydrogen Peroxide Levels in Arabidopsis thaliana and Oilseed Rape Spring Variety Brassica napus L. cv. Mozart(F). J Integr Plant Biol. 2012 Aug;54(8):540-54.

[66] Balazadeh S, Kwasniewski M, Caldana C, Mehrnia M, Zanor MI, Xue GP, et al. ORS1, an H(2)O(2)-responsive NAC transcription factor, controls senescence in Arabidopsis thaliana. Molecular plant. 2011 Mar;4(2):346-60.

[67] Wu A, Allu AD, Garapati P, Siddiqui H, Dortay H, Zanor MI, et al. JUNGBRUNNEN1, a reactive oxygen species-responsive NAC transcription factor, regulates longevity in Arabidopsis. Plant Cell. 2012 Feb;24(2):482-506.

[68] Eulgem T, Somssich IE. Networks of WRKY transcription factors in defense signaling. Curr Opin Plant Biol. 2007 Aug;10(4):366-71.

[69] Miao Y, Laun T, Zimmermann P, Zentgraf U. Targets of the WRKY53 transcription factor and its role during leaf senescence in Arabidopsis. Plant Mol Biol. 2004 Aug; 55(6):853-67.

[70] Masclaux-Daubresse C, Chardon F. Exploring nitrogen remobilization for seed filling using natural variation in Arabidopsis thaliana. J Exp Bot. 2011 Mar;62(6):2131-42.

[71] Habash DZ, Bernard S, Schondelmaier J, Weyen J, Quarrie SA. The genetics of nitrogen use in hexaploid wheat: N utilisation, development and yield. Theor Appl Genet. 2007 Feb;114(3):403-19.

[72] Rossato L, Laine P, Ourry A. Nitrogen storage and remobilization in Brassica napus L. during the growth cycle: nitrogen fluxes within the plant and changes in soluble protein patterns. J Exp Bot. 2001 Aug;52(361):1655-63.

[73] Malagoli P, Laine P, Le Deunff E, Rossato L, Ney B, Ourry A. Modeling nitrogen uptake in oilseed rape cv Capitol during a growth cycle using influx kinetics of root nitrate transport systems and field experimental data. Plant Physiol. 2004 Jan;134(1): 388-400.

[74] Beuve N, Rispail N, Laine P, Cliquet JB, Ourry A, Le Deunff E. Putative role of γ -aminobutyric acid (GABA) as a long-distance signal in up-regulation of nitrate uptake in Brassica napus L. Plant, Cell & Environment. 2004;27(8):1035-46.

[75] Roberts IN, Caputo C, Criado MV, Funk C. Senescence-associated proteases in plants. Physiologia Plantarum. 2012 May;145(1):130-9.

[76] Desclos M, Etienne P, Coquet L, Jouenne T, Bonnefoy J, Segura R, et al. A combined N-15 tracing/proteomics study in Brassica napus reveals the chronology of proteomics events associated with N remobilisation during leaf senescence induced by nitrate limitation or starvation. Proteomics. 2009 Jul;9(13):3580-608.

[77] Waditee-Sirisattha R, Shibato J, Rakwal R, Sirisattha S, Hattori A, Nakano T, et al. The Arabidopsis aminopeptidase LAP2 regulates plant growth, leaf longevity and stress response. The New phytologist. 2011 Sep;191(4):958-69.

[78] Martinez M, Cambra I, Gonzalez-Melendi P, Santamaria ME, Diaz I. C1A cysteine-proteases and their inhibitors in plants. Physiologia Plantarum. 2012 May;145(1): 85-94.

[79] Kmiec B, Glaser E. A novel mitochondrial and chloroplast peptidasome, PreP. Physiologia Plantarum. 2012 May;145(1):180-6.

[80] Lin J-F, Wu S-H. Molecular events in senescing Arabidopsis leaves. The Plant Journal. 2004;39(4):612-28.

[81] Wagner R, Aigner H, Funk C. FtsH proteases located in the plant chloroplast. Physiol Plant. 2011 May;145(1):203-14.

[82] Clarke AK. The chloroplast ATP-dependent Clp protease in vascular plants – new dimensions and future challenges. Physiologia Plantarum. 2011;145(1):235-44.

[83] Haussuhl K, Andersson B, Adamska I. A chloroplast DegP2 protease performs the primary cleavage of the photodamaged D1 protein in plant photosystem II. EMBO J. 2001 Feb 15;20(4):713-22.

[84] Chauhan S, Srivalli S, Nautiyal AR, Khanna-Chopra R. Wheat cultivars differing in heat tolerance show a differential response to monocarpic senescence under high-temperature stress and the involvement of serine proteases. Photosynthetica. 2009 Dec;47(4):536-47.

[85] Parrott DL, McInnerney K, Feller U, Fischer AM. Steam-girdling of barley (Hordeum vulgare) leaves leads to carbohydrate accumulation and accelerated leaf senescence, facilitating transcriptomic analysis of senescence-associated genes. New Phytologist. 2007;176(1):56-69.

[86] Peoples MB, Dalling MJ. The interplay between proteolysis and amino acid metabolism during senescence and nitrogen reallocation. In: Senescence and Aging in Plants, LD Nooden and AC Leopold (eds), pp 181-217. 1988.

[87] Reumann S, Voitsekhovskaja O, Lillo C. From signal transduction to autophagy of plant cell organelles: lessons from yeast and mammals and plant-specific features. Protoplasma. 2010 Dec;247(3-4):233-56.

[88] Hörtensteiner S. Chlorophyll degradation during senescence. Annu Rev Plant Biol. 2006;57:55-77.

[89] Martínez DE, Costa ML, Gomez FM, Otegui MS, Guiamet JJ. 'Senescence-associated vacuoles' are involved in the degradation of chloroplast proteins in tobacco leaves. The Plant Journal. 2008;56(2):196-206.

[90] Feller U, Anders I, Mae T. Rubiscolytics: fate of Rubisco after its enzymatic function in a cell is terminated. Journal of Experimental Botany. 2008 May 1, 2008;59(7): 1615-24.

[91] Kokubun N, Ishida H, Makino A, Mae T. The Degradation of the Large Subunit of Ribulose-1,5-bisphosphate Carboxylase/oxygenase into the 44-kDa Fragment in the

Lysates of Chloroplasts Incubated in Darkness. Plant and Cell Physiology. 2002 November 15, 2002;43(11):1390-5.

[92] Kato Y, Murakami S, Yamamoto Y, Chatani H, Kondo Y, Nakano T, et al. The DNA-binding protease, CND41, and the degradation of ribulose-1,5-bisphosphate carboxylase/oxygenase in senescent leaves of tobacco. Planta. 2004 Nov;220(1):97-104.

[93] Kato Y, Yamamoto Y, Murakami S, Sato F. Post-translational regulation of CND41 protease activity in senescent tobacco leaves. Planta. 2005 Nov;222(4):643-51.

[94] Nakano T, Nagata N, Kimura T, Sekimoto M, Kawaide H, Murakami S, et al. CND41, a chloroplast nucleoid protein that regulates plastid development, causes reduced gibberellin content and dwarfism in tobacco. Physiologia Plantarum. 2003;117(1):130-6.

[95] Ishida H, Yoshimoto K, Izumi M, Reisen D, Yano Y, Makino A, et al. Mobilization of rubisco and stroma-localized fluorescent proteins of chloroplasts to the vacuole by an ATG gene-dependent autophagic process. Plant Physiol. 2008 Sep;148(1):142-55.

[96] Wada S, Ishida H, Izumi M, Yoshimoto K, Ohsumi Y, Mae T, et al. Autophagy plays a role in chloroplast degradation during senescence in individually darkened leaves. Plant Physiol. 2009 Feb;149(2):885-93.

[97] Ishida H, Nishimori Y, Sugisawa M, Makino A, Mae T. The large subunit of ribulose-1,5-bisphosphate carboxylase/oxygenase is fragmented into 37-kDa and 16-kDa polypeptides by active oxygen in the lysates of chloroplasts from primary leaves of wheat. Plant & cell physiology. 1997 Apr;38(4):471-9.

[98] Otegui MS, Noh YS, Martinez DE, Vila Petroff MG, Staehelin LA, Amasino RM, et al. Senescence-associated vacuoles with intense proteolytic activity develop in leaves of Arabidopsis and soybean. Plant J. 2005 Mar;41(6):831-44.

[99] Büchert AM, Civello PM, Martinez GA. Chlorophyllase versus pheophytinase as candidates for chlorophyll dephytilation during senescence of broccoli. J Plant Physiol. 2011 Mar 1;168(4):337-43.

[100] Hörtensteiner S, Feller U. Nitrogen metabolism and remobilization during senescence. Journal of Experimental Botany. 2002 Apr;53(370):927-37.

[101] Chung DW, Pruzinská A, Hörtensteiner S, Ort DR. The Role of Pheophorbide a Oxygenase Expression and Activity in the Canola Green Seed Problem. Plant Physiology. 2006 September 2006;142(1):88-97.

[102] Matile P, Schellenberg M. The cleavage of phaeophorbide a is located in the envelope of barley gerontoplasts. Plant Physiology and Biochemistry. 1996 Jan-Feb;34(1):55-9.

[103] Guiboileau A, Yoshimoto K, Soulay F, Bataille MP, Avice JC, Masclaux-Daubresse C. Autophagy machinery controls nitrogen remobilization at the whole-plant level under both limiting and ample nitrate conditions in Arabidopsis. New Phytologist. 2012 May;194(3):732-40.

[104] Liu Y, Bassham DC. Autophagy: pathways for self-eating in plant cells. Annu Rev Plant Biol. 2012 Jun 2;63:215-37.

[105] Yoshimoto K. Plant autophagy puts the brakes on cell death by controlling salicylic acid signaling. Autophagy. 2010 Jan;6(1):192-3.

[106] Soudry E, Ulitzur S, Gepstein S. Accumulation and remobilization of amino acids during senescence of detached and attached leaves: in planta analysis of tryptophan levels by recombinant luminescent bacteria. J Exp Bot. 2005 Feb;56(412):695-702.

[107] Martin A, Lee J, Kichey T, Gerentes D, Zivy M, Tatout C, et al. Two Cytosolic Glutamine Synthetase Isoforms of Maize Are Specifically Involved in the Control of Grain Production. The Plant Cell Online. 2006 November 2006;18(11):3252-74.

[108] Kumagai E, Araki T, Hamaoka N, Ueno O. Ammonia emission from rice leaves in relation to photorespiration and genotypic differences in glutamine synthetase activity. Annals of Botany. 2011 September 20, 2011.

[109] Kohl S, Hollmann J, Blattner FR, Radchuk V, Andersch F, Steuernagel B, et al. A putative role for amino acid permeases in sink-source communication of barley tissues uncovered by RNA-seq. BMC plant biology. 2012 Aug 30;12(1):154.

[110] Lam H-M, Wong P, Chan H-K, Yam K-M, Chen L, Chow C-M, et al. Overexpression of the ASN1 Gene Enhances Nitrogen Status in Seeds of Arabidopsis. Plant Physiology. 2003 June 1, 2003;132(2):926-35.

[111] Fan S-C, Lin C-S, Hsu P-K, Lin S-H, Tsay Y-F. The Arabidopsis Nitrate Transporter NRT1.7, Expressed in Phloem, Is Responsible for Source-to-Sink Remobilization of Nitrate. The Plant Cell Online. 2009 September 2009;21(9):2750-61.

[112] Khanna-Chopra R. Leaf senescence and abiotic stresses share reactive oxygen species-mediated chloroplast degradation. Protoplasma. 2012 Jul;249(3):469-81.

[113] Queval G, Jaillard D, Zechmann B, Noctor G. Increased intracellular H(2)O(2) availability preferentially drives glutathione accumulation in vacuoles and chloroplasts. Plant Cell Environ. 2011 Jan;34(1):21-32.

[114] Apel K, Hirt H. Reactive oxygen species: metabolism, oxidative stress, and signal transduction. Annu Rev Plant Biol. 2004;55:373-99.

[115] Foyer CH, Noctor G. Redox Homeostasis and Antioxidant Signaling: A Metabolic Interface between Stress Perception and Physiological Responses. The Plant Cell Online. 2005 July 2005;17(7):1866-75.

[116] Noctor G, Foyer CH. ASCORBATE AND GLUTATHIONE: Keeping Active Oxygen Under Control. Annu Rev Plant Physiol Plant Mol Biol. 1998 Jun;49:249-79.

[117] Foyer CH, Noctor G. Ascorbate and Glutathione: The Heart of the Redox Hub. Plant Physiology. 2011 January 1, 2011;155(1):2-18.

[118] Asada K. Production and Scavenging of Reactive Oxygen Species in Chloroplasts and Their Functions. Plant Physiology. 2006 June 2006;141(2):391-6.

[119] Asada K. The Water-Water Cycle in Chloroplasts: Scavenging of Active Oxygens and Dissipation of Excess Photons. Annu Rev Plant Physiol Plant Mol Biol. 1999 Jun; 50:601-39.

[120] Miller GAD, Suzuki N, Ciftci-Yilmaz S, Mittler RON. Reactive oxygen species homeostasis and signalling during drought and salinity stresses. Plant, Cell & Environment. 2010;33(4):453-67.

[121] Torres MA, Dangl JL. Functions of the respiratory burst oxidase in biotic interactions, abiotic stress and development. Current Opinion in Plant Biology. 2005;8(4):397-403.

[122] Kwak JM, Mori IC, Pei ZM, Leonhardt N, Torres MA, Dangl JL, et al. NADPH oxidase AtrbohD and AtrbohF genes function in ROS-dependent ABA signaling in Arabidopsis. EMBO J. 2003 Jun 2;22(11):2623-33.

[123] Daudi A, Cheng Z, O'Brien JA, Mammarella N, Khan S, Ausubel FM, et al. The Apoplastic Oxidative Burst Peroxidase in Arabidopsis Is a Major Component of Pattern-Triggered Immunity. The Plant Cell Online. 2012 January 1, 2012;24(1):275-87.

[124] Groppa M, Ianuzzo M, Rosales E, Vázquez S, Benavides M. Cadmium modulates NADPH oxidase activity and expression in sunflower leaves. Biologia Plantarum. 2012;56(1):167-71.

[125] Foreman J, Demidchik V, Bothwell JH, Mylona P, Miedema H, Torres MA, et al. Reactive oxygen species produced by NADPH oxidase regulate plant cell growth. Nature. 2003 Mar 27;422(6930):442-6.

[126] Takahashi S, Kimura S, Kaya H, Iizuka A, Wong HL, Shimamoto K, et al. Reactive oxygen species production and activation mechanism of the rice NADPH oxidase OsRbohB. Journal of Biochemistry. 2012 July 1, 2012;152(1):37-43.

[127] Molassiotis A, Fotopoulos V. Oxidative and nitrosative signaling in plants: two branches in the same tree? Plant Signal Behav. 2011 Feb;6(2):210-4.

[128] Jin CW, Du ST, Shamsi IH, Luo BF, Lin XY. NO synthase-generated NO acts downstream of auxin in regulating Fe-deficiency-induced root branching that enhances Fe-deficiency tolerance in tomato plants. Journal of Experimental Botany. 2011 July 1, 2011;62(11):3875-84.

[129] Hancock JT. NO synthase? Generation of nitric oxide in plants. Period Biol. 2012 Mar; 114(1):19-24.

[130] Lozano-Juste J, León J. Enhanced Abscisic Acid-Mediated Responses in nia1nia2noa1-2 Triple Mutant Impaired in NIA/NR- and AtNOA1-Dependent Nitric Oxide Biosynthesis in Arabidopsis. Plant Physiology. 2010 February 2010;152(2): 891-903.

[131] Guo F-Q, Okamoto M, Crawford NM. Identification of a Plant Nitric Oxide Synthase Gene Involved in Hormonal Signaling. Science. 2003 October 3, 2003;302(5642):100-3.

[132] Zemojtel T, Fröhlich A, Palmieri MC, Kolanczyk M, Mikula I, Wyrwicz LS, et al. Plant nitric oxide synthase: a never-ending story? Trends in Plant Science. 2006;11(11):524-5.

[133] Seligman K, Saviani EE, Oliveira HC, Pinto-Maglio CAF, Salgado I. Floral Transition and Nitric Oxide Emission During Flower Development in Arabidopsis thaliana is Affected in Nitrate Reductase-Deficient Plants. Plant and Cell Physiology. 2008 July 1, 2008;49(7):1112-21.

[134] Modolo LV, Augusto O, Almeida IMG, Magalhaes JR, Salgado I. Nitrite as the major source of nitric oxide production by Arabidopsis thaliana in response to Pseudomonas syringae. FEBS Letters. 2005;579(17):3814-20.

[135] Planchet E, Jagadis Gupta K, Sonoda M, Kaiser WM. Nitric oxide emission from tobacco leaves and cell suspensions: rate limiting factors and evidence for the involvement of mitochondrial electron transport. The Plant Journal. 2005;41(5):732-43.

[136] Rümer S, Gupta KJ, Kaiser WM. Plant cells oxidize hydroxylamines to NO. Journal of Experimental Botany. 2009 May 1, 2009;60(7):2065-72.

[137] Lee S, Seo PJ, Lee HJ, Park CM. A NAC transcription factor NTL4 promotes reactive oxygen species production during drought-induced leaf senescence in Arabidopsis. Plant J. 2012 Jun;70(5):831-44.

[138] Lum HK, Butt YKC, Lo SCL. Hydrogen Peroxide Induces a Rapid Production of Nitric Oxide in Mung Bean (Phaseolus aureus). Nitric Oxide. 2002;6(2):205-13.

[139] Bright J, Desikan R, Hancock JT, Weir IS, Neill SJ. ABA-induced NO generation and stomatal closure in Arabidopsis are dependent on H2O2 synthesis. The Plant Journal. 2006;45(1):113-22.

[140] He J, Xu H, She X, Song X, Zhao W. The role and the interrelationship of hydrogen peroxide and nitric oxide in the UV-B-induced stomatal closure in broad bean. Functional Plant Biology. 2005;32(3):237-47.

[141] Neill S, Barros R, Bright J, Desikan R, Hancock J, Harrison J, et al. Nitric oxide, stomatal closure, and abiotic stress. Journal of Experimental Botany. 2008 February 1, 2008;59(2):165-76.

[142] Malolepsza U, Rózlska S. Nitric oxide and hydrogen peroxide in tomato resistance: Nitric oxide modulates hydrogen peroxide level in o-hydroxyethylorutin-induced resistance to Botrytis cinerea in tomato. Plant Physiology and Biochemistry. 2005;43(6): 623-35.

[143] Kovtun Y, Chiu W-L, Tena G, Sheen J. Functional analysis of oxidative stress-activated mitogen-activated protein kinase cascade in plants. Proceedings of the National Academy of Sciences. 2000 March 14, 2000;97(6):2940-5.

[144] Wang P, Du Y, Li Y, Ren D, Song CP. Hydrogen peroxide-mediated activation of MAP kinase 6 modulates nitric oxide biosynthesis and signal transduction in Arabidopsis. Plant Cell. 2010 Sep;22(9):2981-98.

[145] Aihong L, Wang Y, Tang J, Xue P, Li C, Liu L, et al. Nitric Oxide and Protein S-nitrosylation Are Integral to Hydrogen Peroxide Induced Leaf Cell Death in Rice. Plant Physiology. 2011 November 21, 2011.

[146] Leshem YaY, Wills RBH, Ku VV-V. Evidence for the function of the free radical gas - nitric oxide (NO) - as an endogenous maturation and senescence regulating factor in higher plants. Plant Physiology and Biochemistry. 1998;36(11):825-33.

[147] del Rio LA, Corpas FJ, Barroso JB. Nitric oxide and nitric oxide synthase activity in plants. Phytochemistry. 2004 Apr;65(7):783-92.

[148] Mishina TE, Lamb C, Zeier J. Expression of a nitric oxide degrading enzyme induces a senescence programme in Arabidopsis. Plant, Cell & Environment. 2007;30(1): 39-52.

[149] Beligni MV, Fath A, Bethke PC, Lamattina L, Jones RL. Nitric Oxide Acts as an Antioxidant and Delays Programmed Cell Death in Barley Aleurone Layers. Plant Physiology. 2002 August 1, 2002;129(4):1642-50.

[150] Møller IM, Sweetlove LJ. ROS signalling - specificity is required. Trends in Plant Science. 2010;15(7):370-4.

[151] Moreno J, Garcia-Murria MJ, Marin-Navarro J. Redox modulation of Rubisco conformation and activity through its cysteine residues. J Exp Bot. 2008;59(7):1605-14.

[152] Marin-Navarro J, Moreno J. Cysteines 449 and 459 modulate the reduction-oxidation conformational changes of ribulose 1.5-bisphosphate carboxylase/oxygenase and the translocation of the enzyme to membranes during stress. Plant Cell Environ. 2006 May;29(5):898-908.

[153] Goud PB, Kachole MS. Role of chloroplastidial proteases in leaf senescence. Plant Signal Behav. 2011 Sep;6(9):1371-6.

[154] Zentgraf U, Zimmermann P, Smykowski A. Role of Intracellular Hydrogen Peroxide as Signalling Molecule for Plant Senescence. In: Nagata T, editor. Senescence. Agricultural and Biological Sciences: InTech; 2012.

[155] Miao Y, Laun T, Smykowski A, Zentgraf U. Arabidopsis MEKK1 can take a short cut: it can directly interact with senescence-related WRKY53 transcription factor on the protein level and can bind to its promoter. Plant Molecular Biology. 2007;65(1):63-76.

[156] Miller G, Schlauch K, Tam R, Cortes D, Torres MA, Shulaev V, et al. The Plant NADPH Oxidase RBOHD Mediates Rapid Systemic Signaling in Response to Diverse Stimuli. Sci Signal. 2009 August 18, 2009;2(84):ra45-.

[157] Monshausen GB, Bibikova TN, Messerli MA, Shi C, Gilroy S. Oscillations in extracellular pH and reactive oxygen species modulate tip growth of Arabidopsis root hairs.

Proceedings of the National Academy of Sciences. 2007 December 26, 2007;104(52): 20996-1001.

[158] Mittler R, Vanderauwera S, Suzuki N, Miller G, Tognetti VB, Vandepoele K, et al. ROS signaling: the new wave? Trends in Plant Science. 2011;16(6):300-9.

[159] Derkx AP, Orford S, Griffiths S, Foulkes MJ, Hawkesford MJ. Identification of differentially senescing mutants of wheat and impacts on yield, biomass and nitrogen partitioning(f). J Integr Plant Biol. 2012 Aug;54(8):555-66.

[160] Uauy C, Distelfeld A, Fahima T, Blechl A, Dubcovsky J. A NAC Gene Regulating Senescence Improves Grain Protein, Zinc, and Iron Content in Wheat. Science. 2006 November 24, 2006;314(5803):1298-301.

[161] McAllister CH, Beatty PH, Good AG. Engineering nitrogen use efficient crop plants: the current status. Plant biotechnology journal. 2012 May 18.

Section 4

Immunosenescence and Cancer

Chapter 4

Immunosenescence and Senescence Immunosurveillance: One of the Possible Links Explaining the Cancer Incidence in Ageing Population

Arnaud Augert and David Bernard

Additional information is available at the end of the chapter

http://dx.doi.org/10.5772/55519

1. Introduction

Since the discovery of cellular senescence significant advances were made to understand its molecular determinants and its physiological role in biological processes such as cancer and aging [1]. Recently, an intimate and complex relationship between senescent cells and the immune system has been highlighted [2]. In addition to their role in senescence immunosurveillance, immune cells display altered functions with age. This process is known as immunosenescence. Although immunosenescence is a slightly different mechanism than cellular senescence, it shares some similarities. This review article briefly describes features, markers, triggers and molecular regulators of cellular senescence and focuses on its role during cancer development. We then introduce immunosenescence and highlight what might be its consequences in cancer development. Finally, taking into account that senescence immunosurveillance is crucial for tumor eradication [2], we provide several hypotheses to explain what could be the impact of immunosenescence on senescence immunosurveillance in a specific cancer context.

2. Cellular senescence

2.1. Historical discovery of cellular senescence

Senescence comes from the Latin word *senex* meaning old age. It was observed approximately half a century ago by Leonard Hayflick while cultivating primary human fibroblast [3, 4]. He observed that primary cells proliferate in culture for approximately 55 population doublings before reaching the "Hayflick limit" which marks the end of their proliferative capacity and the entry into an irreversible growth arrest state. He proposed a theory "that the finite lifetime of diploid cells strains *in vitro* may be an expression of ageing or senescence at the cellular level". Since, the term "replicative senescence" has been used to designate this type of cellular senescence but, as we will see, senescence can also be induced in a replicative independent manner in response to various cellular insults. Senescence is not limited to human primary fibroblast as it has been observed in various primary cells [5-8] including immune cells [9] and also takes place in other species such as Mouse [10], Rat [11], Chicken [12], Caenorhabditis elegans [13], Zebrafish [14] and Yeast [15].

2.2. Features of cellular senescence

2.2.1. Morphology

Senescent cells lose their original morphology. Larger than their normal counterparts, they also have a much larger flattened cytoplasm that contain many vacuoles and cytoplasmic filaments [16, 17], a bigger nucleus and nucleoli and are sometimes multinucleated [18, 19]. In some cases, senescent cells display an increase in the number of lysosomes and golgi [20-24].

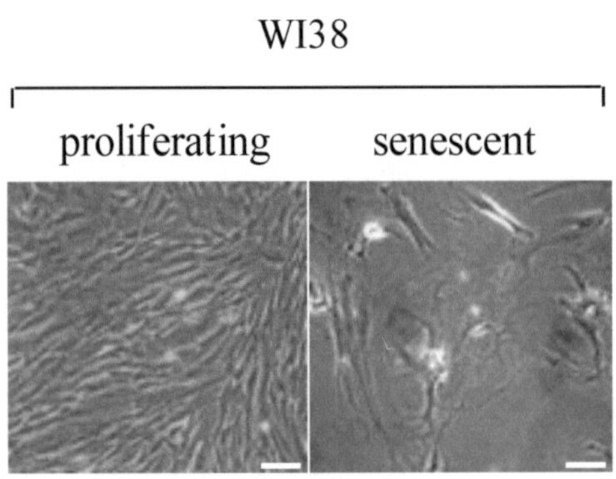

Figure 1. Morphology analysis of primary human fibroblasts (proliferating versus senescent).

2.2.2. Growth arrest

One of the most obvious features of cellular senescence is growth arrest. Indeed, cells are usually blocked in the G1 phase of the cell cycle [25] and in some cases they display (4n) DNA suggesting that cells are either blocked in the late S, G2 or M phases [26, 27]. Cell cycle progression is regulated by cyclin dependent kinases (CDKs) that bind to cyclins [28]. These complexes are regulated by cyclin dependent kinase inhibitors (CKIs) which are essential for the establishment of the senescent growth arrest state [29]. CKIs are divided into two families. The CIP (CDK-interacting protein) and KIP (cyclin-dependent kinase inhibitor protein) [30] and the INK4, for inhibitors of CDK4 [31]. CDK-cyclin complexes favour G1 cell cycle progression by phosphorylating RB family members [32]. RB family proteins are transcriptional co-factors that interact with and inhibit E2F transcription factors activity required for DNA synthesis. Upon the phosphorylation of RB family members by the CDK-type D and E cyclin complexes, E2F transcription factors are released from their interaction with RB proteins leading to cell cycle progression [33] (Figure 2). The CDK4/6-type D cyclins complexes interact with KIP/CIP inhibitors. However, during cellular senescence, INK4 proteins increase and inhibit CDK4/6-cyclin D formation [32]. This enables the activation of RB family members and the inhibition of E2F transcription factors. Additionally, the bioavailability of KIP and CIP proteins increases and they no longer interact with CDK4/6/Cyclin D complexes. It allows them to interact and inhibit CDK2-type E or A cyclin complexes (Figure 2).

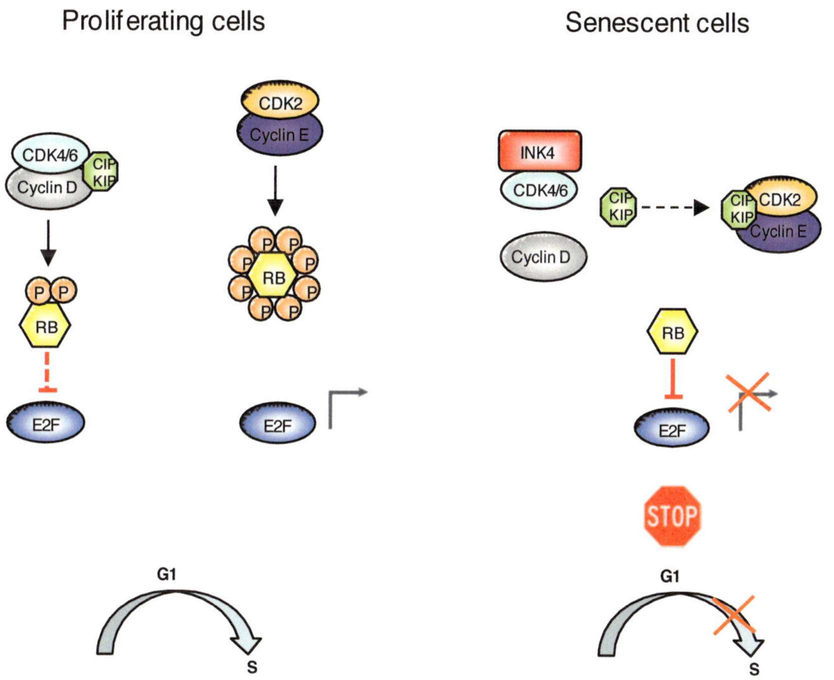

Figure 2. Cell cycle arrest (G1 phase) associated with cellular senescence.

In proliferating cells the CKI levels are low, the CDK/cyclin complexes are functional and RB family members are found hyperphosphorylated leading the E2F family members' activation and G1 progression. In senescent cells, the levels of CKI increase, CDK/Cyclin complexes are inhibited and RB family members are active leading to E2F transcription factors inhibition and G1 cell cycle arrest.

2.2.3. *Altered gene expression*

Senescent cells also display a specific gene expression signature. A notable example are senescence-associated-secretory-phenotype (SASP) molecules such as interleukin 6 (IL-6), interleukin 8 (IL-8), plasminogen activator inhibitor 1 (PAI-1), insulin growth factor binding protein 7 (IGBP7), (ECM) degradation enzymes such as collagenase and metalloprotease (MMPs) but also CKIs, CIP and KIP as previously mentioned [34]. Some genes are also found down-regulated during cellular senescence. It is the case for polycomb complex members such as enhancer of zeste homolog 2 (EZH2) and chromobox homolog 7 (CBX7) [5, 35].

2.2.4. *Senescence markers*

Several markers have been used to specifically identify senescent cells. In addition to an altered cell morphology, growth arrest state and a specific gene expression signature, senescent cells are associated with an increased β-galactosidase activity, detectable at pH 6.0 and known as "senescence-associated-beta-galactosidase (SA-βgal) activity" [36] (Figure 3).

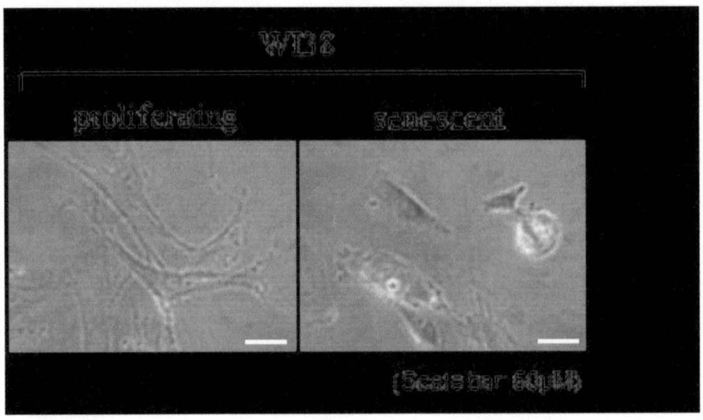

Figure 3. Senescence-associated-beta-galactosidase (SA-βgal) activity detectable at pH6 and yelling a blue colour in senescent cells. Primary human fibroblasts were used for the analysis.

At a chromatin level, specific facultative heterochromatin structures associated with senescent cells were discovered and termed senescence-associated-heterochromatin-foci (SAHF) [37]. These structures regulated by the Retinoblastoma gene (RB) are involved in E2F target genes repression and maintain the cell cycle arrest. They contain markers of heterochromatin such as hypo-acetylated histones, methylated histones (H3K9Me) and the presence of heterochromatin protein 1 (HP1). The histone variant macroH2A, and HMGA a non histone protein, have been identified as crucial regulators in SAHF formation [38] (Figure 4).

2.3. Replicative senescence

Although replicative senescence was first observed in 1961, it took more than 30 years to gain insights into the molecular regulators underlying this process. We now know that it is largely due to telomere lengths and structures. Telomeres are protective structures that cap the end of all eukaryotic chromosomes. They are long double stranded DNA sequences composed of TTAGGG repeats, oriented 5′-to-3′ towards the end of the chromosome (Figure 5) [39]. Telomeres contain a complex composed of six proteins known as the shelterin complex. It comprises telomeric repeat binding factor 1 (TRF1), telomeric repeat binding factor 2 (TRF2), transcriptional repressor/activator protein (RAP1), TRF1-interacting nuclear factor 2 (TIN2),

http://dx.doi.org/10.5772/55519

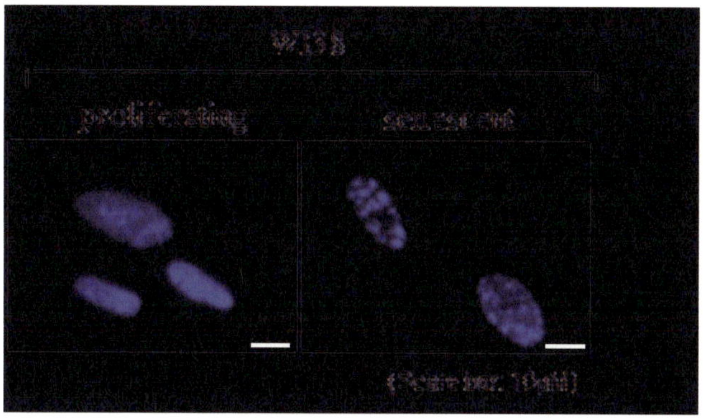

Figure 4. Senescence-associated-heterochromatin-foci (SAHF) of normal and senescent primary human fibroblasts. Dots representing SAHF are visible in senescent cells.

TIN2-interacting protein (TPP1) and protection of telomeres 1 (POT1) (Figure 5). The last two components, TPP1 and POT1 regulate the access of the telomeric substrate for the telomerase [40]. Telomere lengths are maintained by telomerase, a ribonucleoprotein complex that includes a RNA template (known as TERC) and the reverse transcriptase catalytic subunit (TERT) (Figure 5) [40]. Telomerase activity is mainly dictated by the TERT expression, as TERC seems to be ubiquitously transcribed [41]. In 1990, it was noticed that the telomeres length decreased during serially passage human primary fibroblasts and it was suggested that telomere size might be responsible for replicative senescence [42]. Eight years later, it was functionally demonstrated that re-introducing telomerase expression in normal primary cells led to elongated telomeres, lifespan extension and abrogation of replicative senescence [43, 44]. Since then, telomerase re-expression alone [45] or in combination with other alterations [46] has been associated with the immortalisation of various human cells types. Although telomere size is a critical trigger for replicative senescence, telomere structure is also a main determinant [47, 48]. In conclusion, dysfunctional telomeres both short or with an altered structure trigger replicative senescence.

2.4. Premature senescence

2.4.1. Oncogene-induced senescence (OIS)

In 1997, it was observed that in response to an oncogenic form of Ras (H-Ras^{G12V}) primary cells entered a premature senescence state [50]. Oncogene-induced senescence (OIS) is not restricted to Ras but can be extended to most of the MAPK pathway actors (Raf, Mek) and other oncogenic pathways. In accordance, the loss of bona fide tumour suppressors genes that restrain the activity of oncogenic pathways, such as phosphatase and tensin homolog (PTEN), Retinoblastoma (Rb), von Hippel-Lindau tumor suppressor (VHL) and neurofibromin 1 (NF1), has also been associated with premature senescence [10]. OIS is suggested to be a replicative senescence independent mechanism as cells expressing the catalytic subunit of the telomerase (TERT) still undergo OIS [51]. Whereas senescence in ageing tissues had been observed since 1995 [36], the

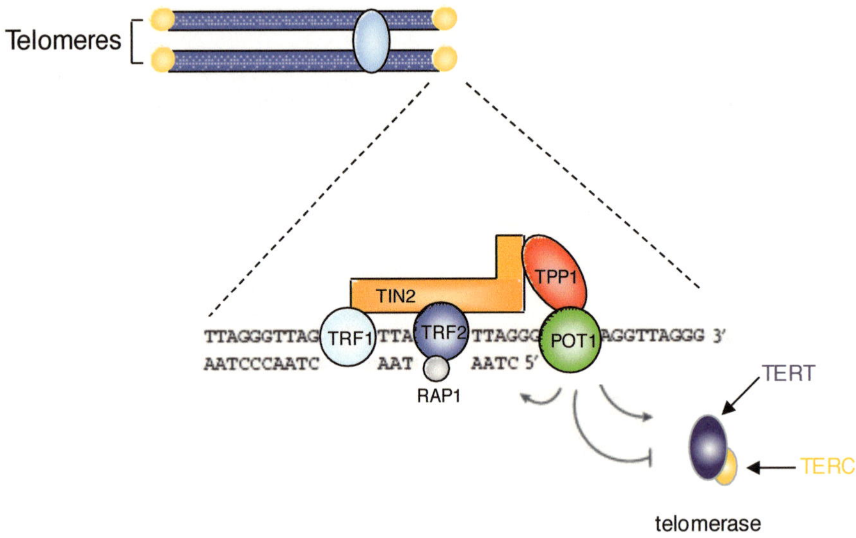

Figure 5. The telomeres and the telomerase. Telomeres, TTAGGG repeats, oriented 5' to 3' towards the end of the chromosome are regulated by six proteins that make up the shelterin complex. The telomeres lengths are maintained by the telomerase, a ribonucleoprotein complex composed of a RNA template (TERC) and the reverse transcriptase catalytic subunit (TERT). Adapted from [49].

demonstration of OIS in a physiological setting was demonstrated ten years later using various mouse model expressing a hyper-active oncogene form or a deleted tumor suppressor [10].

2.4.2. *Oncogene-inactivation-induced senescence (OIIS)*

Cellular senescence is not limited to primary cells but can also be triggered in cancer cells [52]. Cancer cells develop oncogene addiction, a term to describe a cell dependence on an oncogenic pathway to maintain its tumoral properties [53]. Various groups have been trying to identify these oncogene addictions using synthetic lethal screening [53, 54]. Interestingly, targeting oncogene addiction can result in cellular senescence. For example the inhibition of CDK4, a cyclin dependant kinase involved in cell cycle progression, in K-Ras^{G12V} driven non small cell lung carcinoma is associated with cellular senescence induction [55]. Moreover, the inhibition of several embryonic factors known to exert oncogenic properties (T-box 2 (TBX2), twist homolog 1/2 (TWIST 1/2)) can also result in cellular senescence [56, 57]. Finally c-Myc inhibition, a bHLH-LZ transcription factor involved in several tumoral processes such as proliferation, angiogenesis and cell metabolism [58], can leads to senescence induction in cancer cell lines and also in c-Myc transgenic driven lymphomas or osteosarcomas mouse models [59].

2.4.3. *Stress-induced premature senescence (SIPS)*

Stresses are major determinants of cellular senescence [21]. Even if replicative senescence, OIS and OIIS can also generate similar stresses and could be classified in the stress-induced cellular senescence category, we decided to write a specific section for SIPS. Oxygen is one of the major determinants of stress-induced-premature-senescence (SIPS). Oxygen singlet (O_2) is not toxic for cells however O_2 consumption leads to reactive oxygen species (ROS) [21]. ROS can be classified into two groups. The first group which includes reactive species such as superoxide and hydroxyl radicals is composed of molecules with free radical containing one or more unpaired electrons in their outer molecular orbitals. The second group which includes hydrogen peroxide, ozone, peroxinitrate and hydroxide is composed of non-radical ROS that remain chemically reactive and can be converted to radical ROS [60].

Evidences demonstrating that ROS can trigger cellular senescence are now common. For example, cultivating primary human cells in 3% O_2 levels which is closer to the physiological conditions (normal physiological conditions vary from 1-2% in some parts of the brain, skin, heart and kidney to 14% in the lungs) [61], allowed cells to undergo 20 supplemental populations doublings before reaching replicative senescence [62]. Conversely, raising the oxygen levels over 20% or exposing cells to sublethal doses of ROS such as H_20_2 led to a premature senescence like state [63, 64].

SIPS is not restrained to oxidative stress. It can be induced in response to additional inadequate culturing conditions such as abnormal growth factors, the absence of neighbour cells and extracellular matrix components and inadequate concentrations of nutrients, [45, 65, 66]. Other physical, chemical and cellular stressors such as mitomycin C and ionizing radiation can also trigger SIPS [67].

2.5. Pathways regulating cellular senescence

2.5.1. The INK4B/ARF/INK4A

The INK4B/ARF/INK4A locus encodes three tumour suppressor genes that play critical regulatory roles in cellular senescence [31]. Two of these tumour suppressors, $p15^{INK4B}$ and $p16^{INK4A}$, are cyclin dependent kinase inhibitors (CKIs) that trigger cell cycle arrest by inhibiting CDK4 and CDK6 complexes [34]. ARF, the third gene encoded by the locus, is a critical regulator of the p53 tumour suppressor pathway [68]. ARF and $p16^{INK4A}$ share common exons but are encoded in alternative reading frames leading to the production of unique proteins [31].

Polycomb repressive group complexes (PRCs) play a crucial role in the regulation of the locus [69]. The polycomb family is composed of two repressive complexes PRC1 and PRC2. PRC2 establishes the repressive mark leading to the recruitment of the maintenance polycomb complex PRC1. Various polycomb proteins such as CBX7, CBX8, TBX2, TBX3 and Bmi1 have been functionally implicated in the repression of cellular senescence by inhibiting the INK4B/ARF/INK4A locus [5, 70-72]. To counteract the repressive action of the polycomb complexes, several mechanism are activated during cellular senescence. These include the removal or inhibition of polycomb complexes by MAPKAP [73], by the chromatin remodeling SWI/SNF complex [74] and/or the activation of the INK4B/ARF/INK4A locus by JMJD3 [75, 76] (Figure 6).

Additional regulators of the locus include the stress activated p38MAPKinase. Activated in response to various stresses such as high levels of ROS, dysfunctional telomeres and OIS, it regulates cellular senescence in various contexts [77]. It can activate $p16^{INK4A}$, $p15^{INK4B}$ and ARF

[78]. Although the locus products are mainly regulated by epigenetic mechanism, post-translational modifications can also play a role in their regulation. For example, ARF stability is regulated by the E3 ubiquitin ligase TRIP12/ULF [68] and TGF-β stabilises $p15^{INK4B}$ [79]. $p16^{INKA4}$ is activated in response to UV treatment through the inhibition of a SKP2 related degradation [80].

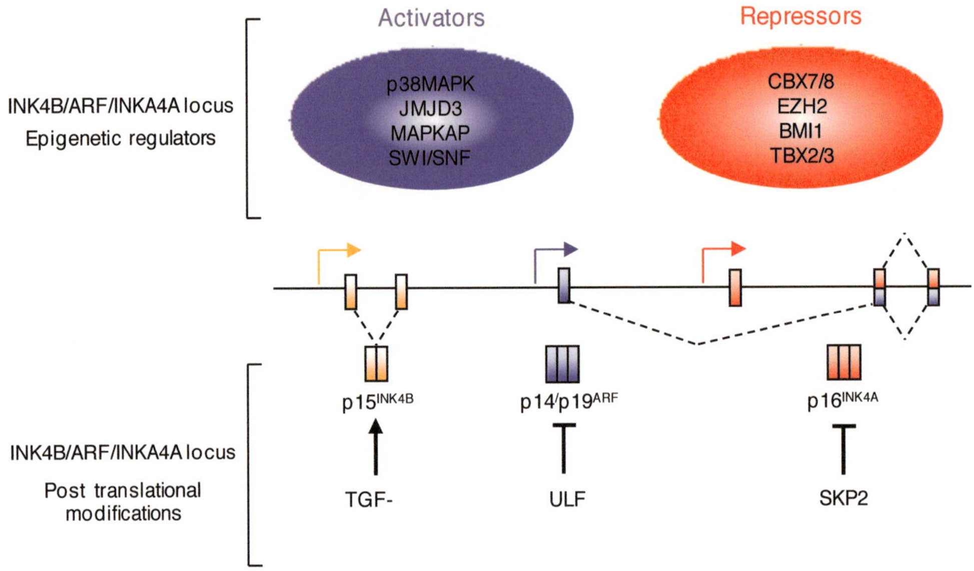

Figure 6. The INK4B/ARF/INK4A locus in cellular senescence.

The locus is mostly regulated by epigenetic mechanism. It involves repressors such as the polycomb proteins (CBX7/8, EZH2, BMI1 and TBX2/3) and activators including histone demethylases (JMJD3), protein kinases (p38MAPK, MAPKAP) and chromatin remodeling complexes (SWI/SNF). Post translational modifications also regulate the locus products.

2.5.2. The DNA damage/p53 pathway

Activated in response to stimuli that trigger a DDR such as dysfunctional telomeres, OIS, ionising radiation and ROS, the p53 pathway is critical in the regulation of senescence [81] (Figure 7).

The activation of a DNA damage response consists in the recruitment of DNA damage sensors at the sites of damage. Various DNA damage sites associated with cellular senescence have been described. These include telomere-dysfunction-induced-foci (TIFs) [82], senescence-associated DNA damage foci (SDF) [83] and DNA segments with chromatin alterations reinforcing senescence (DNA-SCARS) [84].

The DNA damage pathway is activated following the activation of two large protein kinases ataxia-telangiectasia mutated (ATM) and ataxia telangiectasia and Rad3-related (ATR). Once recruited at the DNA damage sites, they phosphorylate and activate the histone variant H2AX [85]. The molecular events involved in single stranded breaks (SSBs) and double stranded breaks (DSBs) then differ and will not be described herein. The activation of the DDR kinases cascade, involving DNA damage mediators and diffusible kinases, results in the phosphorylation and activation of p53 which in turn activates $p21^{CIP1}$, one of its transcriptional targets to regulate growth arrest and cellular senescence [81]. The functional role of DDR in cellular senescence has been demonstrated using various functional approaches. Inactivating DDR proteins as well as p53 and its transcriptional target $p21^{CIP1}$ is sufficient to abrogate cellular senescence in various settings [81]. The p53 pathway can also be activated in a DDR independent mechanism. For example, ARF plays a crucial role in the activation of p53. Activated in response to oncogenic stimulations, it activates p53 by sequestering the E3 ubiquitin protein ligase mouse double minute 2 (MDM2 or HDM2 in humans), an inhibitor of p53 [86] (Figure 7).

The DNA damage/p53 pathway is activated in response to dysfunctional telomeres, oncogenic or oxidative stress, ionizing radiations and cytotoxic drugs. A DNA damage response (DDR) is elicited leading to the activation of local apical kinases, DNA-damage mediators, diffusible kinases and ultimately p53 and $p21^{CIP1}$. The p53 pathway can also be activated by ARF following an oncogenic stress. Adapted from [81].

2.5.3. Reactive oxygen species (ROS)

ROS are critical regulators of OIS [87]. In accordance, ROS regulated proteins such as seladin-1 (modulators of peroxiredoxines, a class of antioxidants) have also been involved in OIS [88]. Enzymes that generate ROS such as 5-lipooxygenase (5LO) mediate Ras induced senescence [89]. ROS are not only involved in Ras induced senescence. Akt was recently identified as a major determinant of various types of cellular senescence by modulating oxygen consumption and down-regulating ROS scavengers [90]. ROS can also mediate replicative senescence. For example, large amount of ROS produced by dysfunctional mitochondria can modulate telomere length and replicative senescence [91]. In accordance, antioxidant proteins can negatively regulate cellular senescence. The extracellular superoxide dismutase (SOD) increases the lifespan of primary cells [92] and over-expressing the antioxidant enzyme catalase to the mitochondria increase mice lifespan [93].

2.5.4. Small non coding RNAs

miRNAs are small (approximately 23 nucleotides) RNAs that play a crucial role in gene regulation [94]. miRNAs bind 3'UTR and sometimes 5'UTR of the mRNA to modulate their translation and/or stability. The regulatory role of miRNAs during cellular senescence has recently been addressed [95]. Expression profiling studies indicate an altered expression among various miRNAs during cellular senescence [95]. Functionally, several miRNAs have been identified as repressor [96] or activators of cellular senescence [97] in normal but also cancer cells [98].

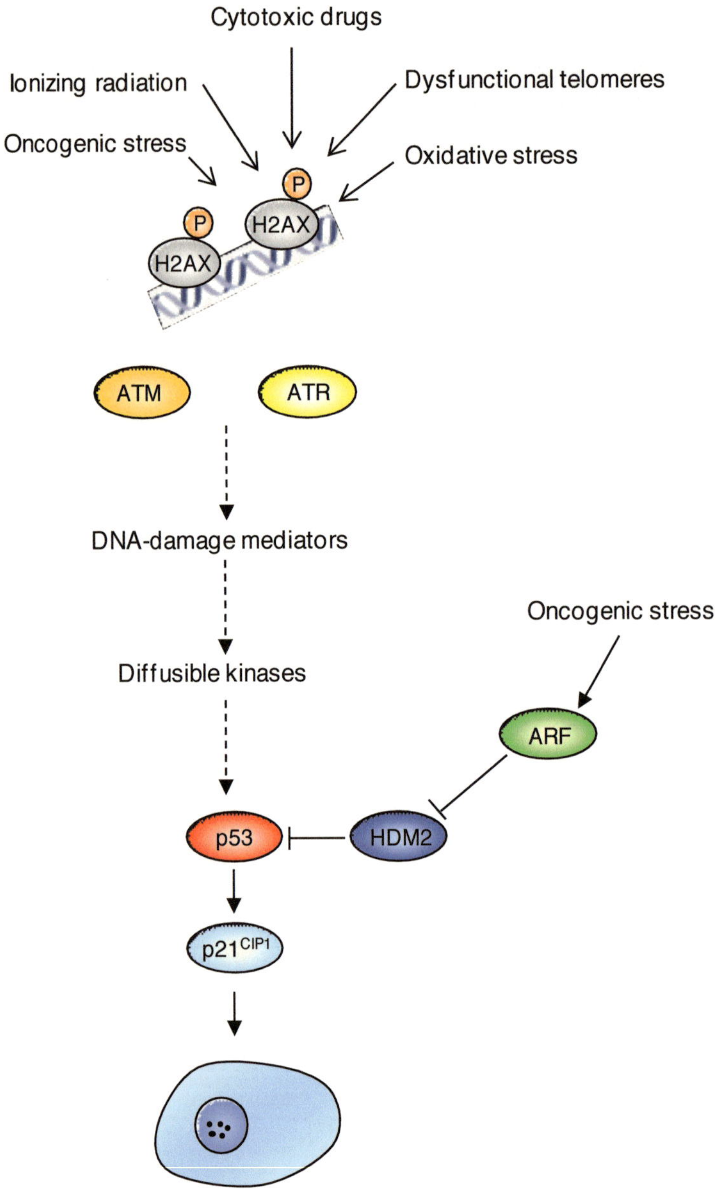

Figure 7. The DNA damage/p53 pathway in cellular senescence.

2.5.5. The autophagic pathway

Autophagy is a recycling process mediated by autophagosomes, which are double membrane vesicules that engulf cytoplasmic contents and then fuse and deliver their content to lysosomes. Lysosomes contain hydrolases that digest the material which ultimately leads to a breakdown of the vesicules and their constituents [99].

Senescent cells display an increase in autophagic vacuoles, a gradual shift from the proteasome pathway to autophagy for polyubiquitinated protein degradation [100] and an upregulation of autophagy regulators such as the ATG related genes (ULK1 and ULK3) [101]. Modulating critical components of the autophagic process can regulate cellular senescence. Inhibition of ATG proteins (ATG-5 and ATG-7) is sufficient to induce an escape from cellular senescence [101]. Conversely, over-expressing ATG target genes such as of ULK3 reduces cell growth [101].

2.6. Cellular senescence and cancer: The tumour point of view

Ever since the discovery and the term replicative senescence introduced by Hayflick in 1965 [3], it has been proposed that senescence can block tumour progression. Primary normal cells are said to be "mortal", and in contrast, cancer cell lines are immortal. Therefore, an escape from replicative senescence is a critical stage that has to be overcome during tumour progression. To physiologically demonstrate this hypothesis, mouse models knockout for the RNA component of the telomerase (TERC$^{-/-}$) were used. The replicative senescence triggered in response to dysfunctional telomeres in these mice was shown to limit tumour progression and lead to tumour regression [102, 103]. In accordance with these results, late generation TERC$^{-/-}$ deficient mice have been shown to be resistant to multistage skin carcinogenesis [104] and are more resistant to tumour formation in a subset of cancer mouse models [105, 106]. Oncogene-induced senescence (OIS) has also been identified as a failsafe program *in vivo,* and this, in response to a physiological aberrant oncogenic activation [10]. Additional inactivation of tumour suppressor genes regulating cellular senescence leads to progression towards malignant stages and full blown tumours [10]. In accordance, premalignant tumour display high levels of senescence whereas it is absent in later stages of tumorigenesis [10]. Finally, cellular senescence is not only a barrier against early stages of tumor progression. It can be reactivated in established tumors leading to tumor eradication [52].

In response to various cellular stresses such as dysfunctional telomeres, oncogene activation, oxidative stress and cytotoxic stresses normal cells acquire various alterations. Cellular senescence is activated to restrain neoplastic expansion. The inactivation of critical tumor suppressor genes (p53, p16^{INK4}, ARF...) leads to cellular senescence escape and progression towards more aggressive tumors. Cellular senescence can be reactivated in tumors in response to the activation of tumor suppressors or oncogene inhibition. This reactivation leads to tumor regression [52].

3. Immunosenescence

3.1. Features of immunosenescence

Cellular senescence can also be detected in immune cells [107]. Immunosenescence is a slightly different process than cellular senescence. Indeed, immunosenescence refers to cellular hypoproliferation in response to mitogenic or antigen stimulation and is often observed in ageing immune cells. In contrast, cellular senescence is associated with a permanent cell cycle arrest underlined with specific molecular markers. Immunosenescence affects both adaptative

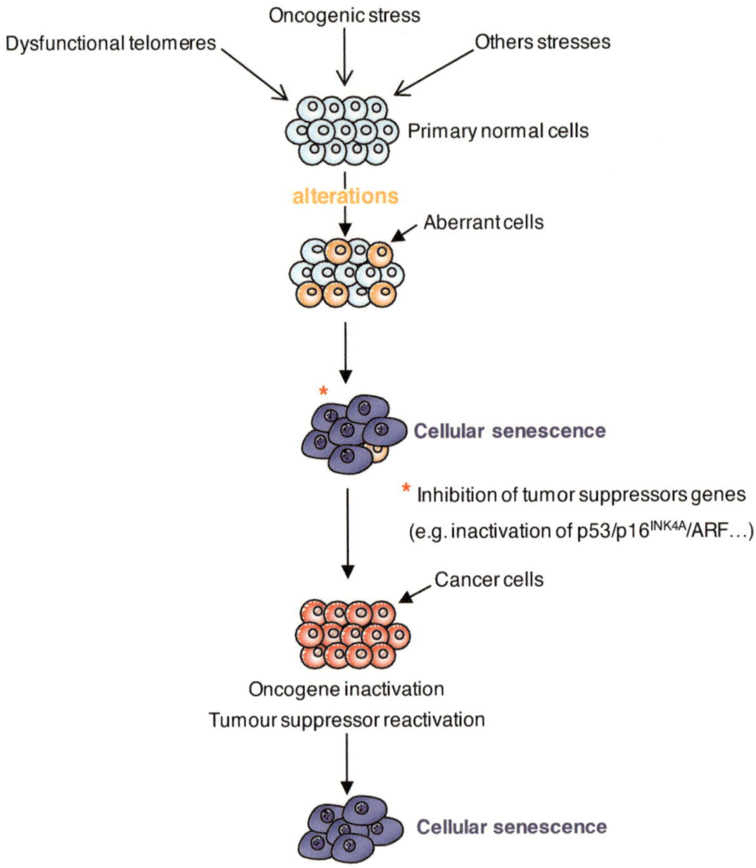

Figure 8. Cellular senescence acts as a tumor suppressive mechanism.

(T and B Lymphocytes) and innate immune cells (Natural killer cells (NK), Natural killer T cells (NKT), Macrophages, Neutrophils, Monocytes and Dendritic cells) [108, 109]. To date, the molecular determinants of immunosenescence have not been very well described. However, similarities with senescence in non immune cells are found. For example, immunosenescence of T cells is regulated by $p16^{INK4A}$ and $p21^{CIP1}$ [110, 111]. Differentiated T cells have shorter telomeres and an inactive telomerase [107]. Functionally, the ectopic telomerase expression maintains telomere size and delays immunosenescence [107]. However, immunosenescence also differs from cellular senescence. For example, inhibiting TNF-α receptor 1 partially reverses T cell immunosenescence in what is suggested to be a caspase-3 dependent mechanism [112]. Specific immunosenescence markers also exist. For example, cell surface markers such as CD27 and CD28 are lost in differentiated senescent CD4+ and CD8+ T cells and the killer cell lectin-like receptor subfamily G member 1 (KLRG1) is also known as a cell surface marker of immunosenescence [107]. Premature immunosenescence has not been characterized so far but one might expect that similar mechanism could be involved in premature senescence and premature immunosenescence. It could be interesting to assess whether stresses such as high ROS levels, chemical or physical cellular stressors can trigger premature senescence. Additionally, it would be interesting to determine if the autophagic pathway and miRNAs are also implicated in various immunosenescence settings.

3.2. The triggers of immunosenescence

Various factors could explain immunosenescence. Thymic involution might play a role. It consists of shrinkage of the thymus with age and results in a decrease output of naïve T lymphocytes [113]. Altered immune signaling also seems to play a role. For example, in the elderly, the composition of lipid rafts is altered and this is associated with a decreased activity of some signaling pathways [114]. Above all, chronic antigen stimulation (e.g. chronic infections, tumor antigens) is the major trigger of immunosenescence. Cytomegalovirus (CMV) but also Epstein-Barr Virus (EBV) infection, to a lesser extent, are determinants of immunosenescence [115]. In accordance, the number of CD8+ cells expressing T cell receptor (TCR) specific CMV antigens in the ageing population increases. This has no effect in the number of T cell in the periphery however the expansion of CMV specific T cells results in a decrease in T cell repertoire [115]. In innate immune cells, an alteration of various receptors activity (e.g. Toll like receptor (TLR)) and in the number of some circulating innate immune cells seem to favor innate immunosenescence [109].

3.3. The consequences of immunosenescence

Immunosenescence is associated with decreased immune functions [109]. Neutrophils, the first innate immune cell to be at the site of pathogen entry, display a decreased chemotaxis and in free radical production and a decreased intracellular killing. Monocytes and macrophages both exhibit a decreased in phagocytosis and NK cells a decreased cytotoxicity. Dendritic cells display decreased phagocytosis, chemotaxis but also a reduced ability to activate the adaptative immune cells via antigen presentation [109]. Additionally to not being efficiently activated by the innate immune cells, adaptative immune cells are also affected by immunosenescence (particularly the T cell compartment). An inhibition of interleukine-2 (IL-2) production, increased DNA damage, telomere shortening but also a decrease in the number of naïve T cell (both CD4+ and CD8+) and an increase in the number of memory T cell leading to a weaker immunosurveillance are observed [115].

4. Immunosenescence and cancer

4.1. Tumors evade the immune system

Escape from immunosurveillance is now considered a cancer hallmark [116]. Immunosurveillance is a term used to define how immune cells identify and destroy abnormal antigen upon recognition [117]. This immunological process required for clearing tumors is often altered during cancer progression giving place to cancer favoring processes such as immunoselection, immunosubversion and ultimately immunosuppression [115, 117]. During cancer development, a complex crosstalk between the tumor and the immune microenvironment takes place. Premalignant tumors send stress signals to the immune cells activating both innate and adaptative responses. In this context of immunosurveillance, the immune response is highly functional and eliminates surrounding tumors. However, tumor cells activate various mechanisms that allow immunosurveillance escape. These include the secretion of various cytokines, mechanisms to induce T cell apoptosis, anergy of naïve T cells, the activation of myeloid suppressor cells, the physical interaction of tumor cells with T cells, the suppression of NKT cell activities and downregulation of cell surface markers [115]. Immunosurveillance escape leads to a state of "equilibrium" between the tumor and the immune system, a process known as immunoselection. It is named as such because aggressive tumor cells that are capable of co-existing or suppressing the immune system are selected [115]. These cells eventually increase in number and secrete various immunosuppressive molecules (e.g. prostaglandin E2 (PGE2), nitric oxides) [117]. The immune system is therefore critical in suppressing tumor growth and its alteration is required from tumor progression. Interestingly, virtually of all the immune cells involved in immunosurveillance are known to be altered with age [115].

4.2. Cancer arises with age: A role for immunosenescence?

Cancer is a pathology associated with age [118]. Indeed, cancer incidence and prevalence increase with age suggesting an important relationship between the two biological processes [118]. During life, an organism is doomed to accumulate mutations favoring cancer development. The triggers of such mutations include environmental factors such as carcinogens, UV lights, viruses and free radicals among others [116]. On the other hand, cancer can no longer be regarded as a cell autonomous process. Recent advances demonstrate that the microenvironment plays a crucial role in modulating cancer development [116]. Although the role of the immune system in cancer development in ageing population is currently uncertain, it is clear that the immune system is altered with age [115]. As previously mentioned, the immune system is critical for clearing tumors, at least in early stages of tumorigenesis. Additionally, we have seen that immunosenescence is associated with profound immune alterations leading to a decrease in various immune cells activity. The activation of the adaptative immune response by dendritics cells is crucial for the activation of T-cell. Interestingly in the elders, immunosenescence of dendritics cells which impacts various co-receptors leads to a weakened T cell response [115]. The alteration of TLRs could also favor cancer development in ageing populations. Indeed, TLRs are crucial in the activation of innate immune cells. Their alterations leads to a decreased phagocytosis of innate immune cells and renders them less capable of destroying tumors. Ageing populations also have an increase amount of immune suppressive cells such as T regulatory cells that inhibit innate immune cells activity though direct cell-cell interaction. Myeloid derived suppressor cells (MDSC) are composed of a heterogeneous population of innate immune cells that can suppress the activation of CD4+ and CD8+ T cells. Interestingly, MDSC are activated by various anti-inflammatory signals (e.g IL-10, TGF-β) that are found increased in the elderly. Additionally, IDO, an immunosuppressive molecule that inhibits T cells responses, is also found up-regulated in ageing populations. Changes in the immune system that could favor cancer development are not limited to the innate immune cells. With ageing there is a gradual shift of Th1 towards Th2 in the T cells repertoire and this leads to an alteration in the activity of both naïve and cytotoxic lymphocytes. In summary, various immunosuppressive mechanisms are found up-regulated in the elderly [115]. Considering the crucial role of the immune system in cancer eradication, it suggests that immunosenescence could play a role in cancers associated with age.

5. Immunosenescence and senescence immunosurveillance

5.1. Senescence immunosurveillance

An intimate relationship between cellular senescence and the immune system has recently been identified [2]. Using various mouse models, it was demonstrated that the reactivation of p53 in established tumours was associated with cellular senescence and tumour regression [119, 120]. However, as senescent cells do not die of apoptosis and can persist in some tissue for many years [121], the fate of senescent cells remained uncertain especially in a cancer context. Since the discovery of a secretory phenotype associated with cellular senescence (SASP), it has been suggested that senescent cells can initiate cross-talks with the microenvironment [2]. It was therefore hypothesised that senescent cells could be cleared by the immune system. In accordance, it was demonstrated in a mouse model of liver carcinoma that the activation of an innate immune response (NK cells macrophage and neutrophils) was responsible for the clearance of senescent tumours [120]. In liver cancer, senescence immunosurveillance thus seems to be required to clear senescent tumors. Interestingly, senescence immunosurveillance is not limited to liver cancer as it was also required for the complete remission of lymphoma and leukemia mouse models [122]. In these models, the adaptative immune response and more specifically CD4+ T cells were necessary for tumour eradication and also for senescence induction suggesting a complex interplay between senescent cells and the immune system [2]. Such interplay has been tackled in a mouse model of lymphomagenesis [123]. In a model of OIS *in vivo* resulting in apoptosis, macrophage were attracted and required to engulf apoptotic reminders. Both cellular senescence and apoptosis were shown to act together via the innate immune response to inhibit tumour progression. In turn, activated macrophages secreted various cytokines such as TGF-β to induce cellular senescence of malignant cells [123]. These results clearly demonstrate a crucial role of immunosurveillance in clearing senescent tumors and amplifying senescence induction. To reinforce the role of senescence immunosurveillance as a barrier against cancer, the inactivation of CD4+ T cell following OIS of hepatocytes in mice led to tumor progression [124].The role CD4+ T cell in preventing tumor progression in this mouse model was dependent upon the activation of monocytes and macrophages [124]. What is surprising is that the inhibition of cellular senescence did not activate the immune system suggesting that during cancer development a functional senescence response might be required for an efficient immunosurveillance and tumor suppression [125]. It is therefore tempting to suggest that cellular senescence plays a significant role during immunosuppression [126]. It will also be interesting to demonstrate if senescence immunosurveillance also takes place in other organs during cancer development and whether it is involved in tumor suppression.

5.2. Defects in senescence immunosurveillance: A role for immunosenescence?

It appears that a functional immune system is required for efficient senescence clearance and tumor suppression. As immunosenescence affects normal immune homeostasis and senescent cells increase with age [118], it is tempting to speculate that in the elderly a defect in senescence immunosurveillance could contribute to the increased cancer incidence. In line with this hypothesis is the fact that all the immune cells involved in senescence immunosurveillance seem to be altered with age. However, to date no functional experiments have been carried to test such hypothesis. Mouse models of ageing recapitulating immunosenescence in which cellular senescence is induced could be of great interest to determine this possibility.

6. Conclusion

Immunosenescence is a field that holds great promises. To date, some of the molecular determinants of immunosenescence are still to be discovered. Identifying such mechanism could shed light on this cellular process and might help us to find ways to counteract such mechanism. Additionally, assessing the role of immunosenescence during cancer development in ageing population and more specifically its role during senescence immunosurveillance in the elderly could shed light on the mechanism associated with cancer.

Author details

Arnaud Augert and David Bernard

*Address all correspondence to: david.bernard@lyon.unicancer.fr

Centre de Recherche en Cancérologie de Lyon, UMR INSERM U1052/CNRS 5286, Centre Léon Bérard, Université de Lyon, France

References

[1] Collado M, Blasco MA, Serrano M. Cellular senescence in cancer and aging. Cell. 2007 Jul 27;130(2):223-33.

[2] Serrano M. Cancer: final act of senescence. Nature. 2011 Nov 24;479(7374):481-2.

[3] Hayflick L. The Limited in Vitro Lifetime of Human Diploid Cell Strains. Exp Cell Res. 1965 Mar;37:614-36.

[4] Hayflick L, Moorhead PS. The serial cultivation of human diploid cell strains. Exp Cell Res. 1961 Dec;25:585-621.

[5] Gil J, Bernard D, Martinez D, Beach D. Polycomb CBX7 has a unifying role in cellular lifespan. Nat Cell Biol. 2004 Jan;6(1):67-72.

[6] Rheinwald JG, Green H. Serial cultivation of strains of human epidermal keratinocytes: the formation of keratinizing colonies from single cells. Cell. 1975 Nov;6(3): 331-43.

[7] Romanov SR, Kozakiewicz BK, Holst CR, Stampfer MR, Haupt LM, Tlsty TD. Normal human mammary epithelial cells spontaneously escape senescence and acquire genomic changes. Nature. 2001 Feb 1;409(6820):633-7.

[8] Tassin J, Malaise E, Courtois Y. Human lens cells have an in vitro proliferative capacity inversely proportional to the donor age. Exp Cell Res. 1979 Oct 15;123(2): 388-92.

[9] Tice RR, Schneider EL, Kram D, Thorne P. Cytokinetic analysis of the impaired proliferative response of peripheral lymphocytes from aged humans to phytohemagglutinin. J Exp Med. 1979 May 1;149(5):1029-41.

[10] Collado M, Serrano M. Senescence in tumours: evidence from mice and humans. Nat Rev Cancer. 2010 Jan;10(1):51-7.

[11] Melk A, Kittikowit W, Sandhu I, Halloran KM, Grimm P, Schmidt BM, et al. Cell senescence in rat kidneys in vivo increases with growth and age despite lack of telomere shortening. Kidney Int. 2003 Jun;63(6):2134-43.

[12] Kim TW, Kim HJ, Lee C, Kim HY, Baek SH, Kim JH, et al. Identification of replicative senescence-associated genes in human umbilical vein endothelial cells by an annealing control primer system. Exp Gerontol. 2008 Apr;43(4):286-95.

[13] Burks DJ, Font de Mora J, Schubert M, Withers DJ, Myers MG, Towery HH, et al. IRS-2 pathways integrate female reproduction and energy homeostasis. Nature. 2000 Sep 21;407(6802):377-82.

[14] Patton EE, Widlund HR, Kutok JL, Kopani KR, Amatruda JF, Murphey RD, et al. BRAF mutations are sufficient to promote nevi formation and cooperate with p53 in the genesis of melanoma. Curr Biol. 2005 Feb 8;15(3):249-54.

[15] Lundblad V, Szostak JW. A mutant with a defect in telomere elongation leads to senescence in yeast. Cell. 1989 May 19;57(4):633-43.

[16] Comings DE, Okada TA. Electron microscopy of human fibroblasts in tissue culture during logarithmic and confluent stages of growth. Exp Cell Res. 1970 Aug;61(2): 295-301.

[17] Lipetz J, Cristofalo VJ. Ultrastructural changes accompanying the aging of human diploid cells in culture. J Ultrastruct Res. 1972 Apr;39(1):43-56.

[18] Cristofalo VJ, Kritchevsky D. Cell size and nucleic acid content in the diploid human cell line WI-38 during aging. Med Exp Int J Exp Med. 1969;19(6):313-20.

[19] Mitsui Y, Schneider EL. Increased nuclear sizes in senescent human diploid fibroblast cultures. Exp Cell Res. 1976 Jun;100(1):147-52.

[20] Brunk U, Ericsson JL, Ponten J, Westermark B. Residual bodies and "aging" in cultured human glia cells. Effect of entrance into phase 3 and prolonged periods of confluence. Exp Cell Res. 1973 Apr;79(1):1-14.

[21] Cristofalo VJ, Lorenzini A, Allen RG, Torres C, Tresini M. Replicative senescence: a critical review. Mech Ageing Dev. 2004 Oct-Nov;125(10-11):827-48.

[22] Gerland LM, Peyrol S, Lallemand C, Branche R, Magaud JP, Ffrench M. Association of increased autophagic inclusions labeled for beta-galactosidase with fibroblastic aging. Exp Gerontol. 2003 Aug;38(8):887-95.

[23] Kurz DJ, Decary S, Hong Y, Erusalimsky JD. Senescence-associated (beta)-galactosidase reflects an increase in lysosomal mass during replicative ageing of human endothelial cells. J Cell Sci. 2000 Oct;113 (Pt 20):3613-22.

[24] Robbins E, Levine EM, Eagle H. Morphologic changes accompanying senescence of cultured human diploid cells. J Exp Med. 1970 Jun 1;131(6):1211-22.

[25] Di Leonardo A, Linke SP, Clarkin K, Wahl GM. DNA damage triggers a prolonged p53-dependent G1 arrest and long-term induction of Cip1 in normal human fibroblasts. Genes Dev. 1994 Nov 1;8(21):2540-51.

[26] Di Micco R, Fumagalli M, Cicalese A, Piccinin S, Gasparini P, Luise C, et al. Oncogene-induced senescence is a DNA damage response triggered by DNA hyper-replication. Nature. 2006 Nov 30;444(7119):638-42.

[27] Wada T, Joza N, Cheng HY, Sasaki T, Kozieradzki I, Bachmaier K, et al. MKK7 couples stress signalling to G2/M cell-cycle progression and cellular senescence. Nat Cell Biol. 2004 Mar;6(3):215-26.

[28] Malumbres M, Barbacid M. Mammalian cyclin-dependent kinases. Trends Biochem Sci. 2005 Nov;30(11):630-41.

[29] Campisi J, d'Adda di Fagagna F. Cellular senescence: when bad things happen to good cells. Nat Rev Mol Cell Biol. 2007 Sep;8(9):729-40.

[30] Malumbres M, Barbacid M. Cell cycle, CDKs and cancer: a changing paradigm. Nat Rev Cancer. 2009 Mar;9(3):153-66.

[31] Kim WY, Sharpless NE. The regulation of INK4/ARF in cancer and aging. Cell. 2006 Oct 20;127(2):265-75.

[32] Gil J, Peters G. Regulation of the INK4b-ARF-INK4a tumour suppressor locus: all for one or one for all. Nat Rev Mol Cell Biol. 2006 Sep;7(9):667-77.

[33] Burkhart DL, Sage J. Cellular mechanisms of tumour suppression by the retinoblastoma gene. Nat Rev Cancer. 2008 Sep;8(9):671-82.

[34] Kuilman T, Michaloglou C, Mooi WJ, Peeper DS. The essence of senescence. Genes Dev. 2010 Nov 15;24(22):2463-79.

[35] Bracken AP, Kleine-Kohlbrecher D, Dietrich N, Pasini D, Gargiulo G, Beekman C, et al. The Polycomb group proteins bind throughout the INK4A-ARF locus and are dissociated in senescent cells. Genes Dev. 2007 Mar 1;21(5):525-30.

[36] Dimri GP, Lee X, Basile G, Acosta M, Scott G, Roskelley C, et al. A biomarker that identifies senescent human cells in culture and in aging skin in vivo. Proc Natl Acad Sci U S A. 1995 Sep 26;92(20):9363-7.

[37] Narita M, Nunez S, Heard E, Narita M, Lin AW, Hearn SA, et al. Rb-mediated heterochromatin formation and silencing of E2F target genes during cellular senescence. Cell. 2003 Jun 13;113(6):703-16.

[38] Zhang R, Chen W, Adams PD. Molecular dissection of formation of senescence-associated heterochromatin foci. Mol Cell Biol. 2007 Mar;27(6):2343-58.

[39] Blasco MA. Telomeres and human disease: ageing, cancer and beyond. Nat Rev Genet. 2005 Aug;6(8):611-22.

[40] Verdun RE, Karlseder J. Replication and protection of telomeres. Nature. 2007 Jun 21;447(7147):924-31.

[41] Cech TR. Beginning to understand the end of the chromosome. Cell. 2004 Jan 23;116(2):273-9.

[42] Harley CB, Futcher AB, Greider CW. Telomeres shorten during ageing of human fibroblasts. Nature. 1990 May 31;345(6274):458-60.

[43] Bodnar AG, Ouellette M, Frolkis M, Holt SE, Chiu CP, Morin GB, et al. Extension of life-span by introduction of telomerase into normal human cells. Science. 1998 Jan 16;279(5349):349-52.

[44] Vaziri H, Benchimol S. Reconstitution of telomerase activity in normal human cells leads to elongation of telomeres and extended replicative life span. Curr Biol. 1998 Feb 26;8(5):279-82.

[45] Ramirez RD, Morales CP, Herbert BS, Rohde JM, Passons C, Shay JW, et al. Putative telomere-independent mechanisms of replicative aging reflect inadequate growth conditions. Genes Dev. 2001 Feb 15;15(4):398-403.

[46] Kiyono T, Foster SA, Koop JI, McDougall JK, Galloway DA, Klingelhutz AJ. Both Rb/p16INK4a inactivation and telomerase activity are required to immortalize human epithelial cells. Nature. 1998 Nov 5;396(6706):84-8.

[47] Karlseder J, Hoke K, Mirzoeva OK, Bakkenist C, Kastan MB, Petrini JH, et al. The telomeric protein TRF2 binds the ATM kinase and can inhibit the ATM-dependent DNA damage response. PLoS Biol. 2004 Aug;2(8):E240.

[48] Stewart SA, Ben-Porath I, Carey VJ, O'Connor BF, Hahn WC, Weinberg RA. Erosion of the telomeric single-strand overhang at replicative senescence. Nat Genet. 2003 Apr;33(4):492-6.

[49] Deng Q, Liao R, Wu BL, Sun P. High intensity ras signaling induces premature senescence by activating p38 pathway in primary human fibroblasts. J Biol Chem. 2004 Jan 9;279(2):1050-9.

[50] Serrano M, Lin AW, McCurrach ME, Beach D, Lowe SW. Oncogenic ras provokes premature cell senescence associated with accumulation of p53 and p16INK4a. Cell. 1997 Mar 7;88(5):593-602.

[51] Wei S, Wei S, Sedivy JM. Expression of catalytically active telomerase does not prevent premature senescence caused by overexpression of oncogenic Ha-Ras in normal human fibroblasts. Cancer Res. 1999 Apr 1;59(7):1539-43.

[52] Nardella C, Clohessy JG, Alimonti A, Pandolfi PP. Pro-senescence therapy for cancer treatment. Nat Rev Cancer. 2011 11(7):503-11.

[53] Luo J, Solimini NL, Elledge SJ. Principles of cancer therapy: oncogene and non-oncogene addiction. Cell. 2009 Mar 6;136(5):823-37.

[54] Barbie DA, Tamayo P, Boehm JS, Kim SY, Moody SE, Dunn IF, et al. Systematic RNA interference reveals that oncogenic KRAS-driven cancers require TBK1. Nature. 2009 Nov 5;462(7269):108-12.

[55] Puyol M, Martin A, Dubus P, Mulero F, Pizcueta P, Khan G, et al. A synthetic lethal interaction between K-Ras oncogenes and Cdk4 unveils a therapeutic strategy for non-small cell lung carcinoma. Cancer Cell. 2010 Jul 13;18(1):63-73.

[56] Ansieau S, Bastid J, Doreau A, Morel AP, Bouchet BP, Thomas C, et al. Induction of EMT by twist proteins as a collateral effect of tumor-promoting inactivation of premature senescence. Cancer Cell. 2008 Jul 8;14(1):79-89.

[57] Vance KW, Carreira S, Brosch G, Goding CR. Tbx2 is overexpressed and plays an important role in maintaining proliferation and suppression of senescence in melanomas. Cancer Res. 2005 Mar 15;65(6):2260-8.

[58] Pelengaris S, Khan M, Evan G. c-MYC: more than just a matter of life and death. Nat Rev Cancer. 2002 Oct;2(10):764-76.

[59] Wu CH, van Riggelen J, Yetil A, Fan AC, Bachireddy P, Felsher DW. Cellular senescence is an important mechanism of tumor regression upon c-Myc inactivation. Proc Natl Acad Sci U S A. 2007 Aug 7;104(32):13028-33.

[60] Trachootham D, Alexandre J, Huang P. Targeting cancer cells by ROS-mediated mechanisms: a radical therapeutic approach? Nat Rev Drug Discov. 2009 Jul;8(7):579-91.

[61] Vaupel P, Kallinowski F, Okunieff P. Blood flow, oxygen and nutrient supply, and metabolic microenvironment of human tumors: a review. Cancer Res. 1989 Dec 1;49(23):6449-65.

[62] Chen Q, Fischer A, Reagan JD, Yan LJ, Ames BN. Oxidative DNA damage and senescence of human diploid fibroblast cells. Proc Natl Acad Sci U S A. 1995 May 9;92(10): 4337-41.

[63] Alaluf S, Muir-Howie H, Hu HL, Evans A, Green MR. Atmospheric oxygen accelerates the induction of a post-mitotic phenotype in human dermal fibroblasts: the key protective role of glutathione. Differentiation. 2000 Oct;66(2-3):147-55.

[64] Horikoshi T, Balin AK, Carter DM. Effects of oxygen tension on the growth and pigmentation of normal human melanocytes. J Invest Dermatol. 1991 Jun;96(6):841-4.

[65] Bennett DC, Medrano EE. Molecular regulation of melanocyte senescence. Pigment Cell Res. 2002 Aug;15(4):242-50.

[66] Loo DT, Fuquay JI, Rawson CL, Barnes DW. Extended culture of mouse embryo cells without senescence: inhibition by serum. Science. 1987 Apr 10;236(4798):200-2.

[67] Toussaint O, Dumont P, Remacle J, Dierick JF, Pascal T, Frippiat C, et al. Stress-induced premature senescence or stress-induced senescence-like phenotype: one in vivo reality, two possible definitions? ScientificWorldJournal. 2002 Jan 29;2:230-47.

[68] Collado M, Serrano M. The TRIP from ULF to ARF. Cancer Cell. 2010 Apr 13;17(4): 317-8.

[69] Popov N, Gil J. Epigenetic regulation of the INK4b-ARF-INK4a locus: in sickness and in health. Epigenetics. 2010 Nov-Dec;5(8):685-90.

[70] Brummelkamp TR, Kortlever RM, Lingbeek M, Trettel F, MacDonald ME, van Lohuizen M, et al. TBX-3, the gene mutated in Ulnar-Mammary Syndrome, is a negative regulator of p19ARF and inhibits senescence. J Biol Chem. 2002 Feb 22;277(8):6567-72.

[71] Jacobs JJ, Keblusek P, Robanus-Maandag E, Kristel P, Lingbeek M, Nederlof PM, et al. Senescence bypass screen identifies TBX2, which represses Cdkn2a (p19(ARF)) and is amplified in a subset of human breast cancers. Nat Genet. 2000 Nov;26(3): 291-9.

[72] Jacobs JJ, Kieboom K, Marino S, DePinho RA, van Lohuizen M. The oncogene and Polycomb-group gene bmi-1 regulates cell proliferation and senescence through the ink4a locus. Nature. 1999 Jan 14;397(6715):164-8.

[73] Voncken JW, Niessen H, Neufeld B, Rennefahrt U, Dahlmans V, Kubben N, et al. MAPKAP kinase 3pK phosphorylates and regulates chromatin association of the polycomb group protein Bmi1. J Biol Chem. 2005 Feb 18;280(7):5178-87.

[74] Kia SK, Gorski MM, Giannakopoulos S, Verrijzer CP. SWI/SNF mediates polycomb eviction and epigenetic reprogramming of the INK4b-ARF-INK4a locus. Mol Cell Biol. 2008 May;28(10):3457-64.

[75] Agger K, Cloos PA, Rudkjaer L, Williams K, Andersen G, Christensen J, et al. The H3K27me3 demethylase JMJD3 contributes to the activation of the INK4A-ARF locus in response to oncogene- and stress-induced senescence. Genes Dev. 2009 May 15;23(10):1171-6.

[76] Barradas M, Anderton E, Acosta JC, Li S, Banito A, Rodriguez-Niedenfuhr M, et al. Histone demethylase JMJD3 contributes to epigenetic control of INK4a/ARF by oncogenic RAS. Genes Dev. 2009 May 15;23(10):1177-82.

[77] Wagner EF, Nebreda AR. Signal integration by JNK and p38 MAPK pathways in cancer development. Nat Rev Cancer. 2009 Aug;9(8):537-49.

[78] Wong ES, Le Guezennec X, Demidov ON, Marshall NT, Wang ST, Krishnamurthy J, et al. p38MAPK controls expression of multiple cell cycle inhibitors and islet proliferation with advancing age. Dev Cell. 2009 Jul;17(1):142-9.

[79] Sandhu C, Garbe J, Bhattacharya N, Daksis J, Pan CH, Yaswen P, et al. Transforming growth factor beta stabilizes p15INK4B protein, increases p15INK4B-cdk4 complexes, and inhibits cyclin D1-cdk4 association in human mammary epithelial cells. Mol Cell Biol. 1997 May;17(5):2458-67.

[80] Al-Khalaf HH, Hendrayani SF, Aboussekhra A. The atr protein kinase controls UV-dependent upregulation of p16INK4A through inhibition of Skp2-related polyubiquitination/degradation. Mol Cancer Res. Mar;9(3):311-9.

[81] d'Adda di Fagagna F. Living on a break: cellular senescence as a DNA-damage response. Nat Rev Cancer. 2008 Jul;8(7):512-22.

[82] Takai H, Smogorzewska A, de Lange T. DNA damage foci at dysfunctional telomeres. Curr Biol. 2003 Sep 2;13(17):1549-56.

[83] d'Adda di Fagagna F, Reaper PM, Clay-Farrace L, Fiegler H, Carr P, Von Zglinicki T, et al. A DNA damage checkpoint response in telomere-initiated senescence. Nature. 2003 Nov 13;426(6963):194-8.

[84] Rodier F, Coppe JP, Patil CK, Hoeijmakers WA, Munoz DP, Raza SR, et al. Persistent DNA damage signalling triggers senescence-associated inflammatory cytokine secretion. Nat Cell Biol. 2009 Aug;11(8):973-9.

[85] Celeste A, Petersen S, Romanienko PJ, Fernandez-Capetillo O, Chen HT, Sedelnikova OA, et al. Genomic instability in mice lacking histone H2AX. Science. 2002 May 3;296(5569):922-7.

[86] Weber JD, Taylor LJ, Roussel MF, Sherr CJ, Bar-Sagi D. Nucleolar Arf sequesters Mdm2 and activates p53. Nat Cell Biol. 1999 May;1(1):20-6.

[87] Lee AC, Fenster BE, Ito H, Takeda K, Bae NS, Hirai T, et al. Ras proteins induce senescence by altering the intracellular levels of reactive oxygen species. J Biol Chem. 1999 Mar 19;274(12):7936-40.

[88] Wu C, Miloslavskaya I, Demontis S, Maestro R, Galaktionov K. Regulation of cellular response to oncogenic and oxidative stress by Seladin-1. Nature. 2004 Dec 2;432(7017):640-5.

[89] Catalano A, Rodilossi S, Caprari P, Coppola V, Procopio A. 5-Lipoxygenase regulates senescence-like growth arrest by promoting ROS-dependent p53 activation. Embo J. 2005 Jan 12;24(1):170-9.

[90] Nogueira V, Park Y, Chen CC, Xu PZ, Chen ML, Tonic I, et al. Akt determines replicative senescence and oxidative or oncogenic premature senescence and sensitizes cells to oxidative apoptosis. Cancer Cell. 2008 Dec 9;14(6):458-70.

[91] Passos JF, Saretzki G, Ahmed S, Nelson G, Richter T, Peters H, et al. Mitochondrial dysfunction accounts for the stochastic heterogeneity in telomere-dependent senescence. PLoS Biol. 2007 May;5(5):e110.

[92] Serra V, von Zglinicki T, Lorenz M, Saretzki G. Extracellular superoxide dismutase is a major antioxidant in human fibroblasts and slows telomere shortening. J Biol Chem. 2003 Feb 28;278(9):6824-30.

[93] Schriner SE, Linford NJ, Martin GM, Treuting P, Ogburn CE, Emond M, et al. Extension of murine life span by overexpression of catalase targeted to mitochondria. Science. 2005 Jun 24;308(5730):1909-11.

[94] Bartel DP. MicroRNAs: target recognition and regulatory functions. Cell. 2009 Jan 23;136(2):215-33.

[95] Liu FJ, Wen T, Liu L. MicroRNAs as a novel cellular senescence regulator. Ageing Res Rev. 2011 Jun 13.

[96] Voorhoeve PM, le Sage C, Schrier M, Gillis AJ, Stoop H, Nagel R, et al. A genetic screen implicates miRNA-372 and miRNA-373 as oncogenes in testicular germ cell tumors. Cell. 2006 Mar 24;124(6):1169-81.

[97] He L, He X, Lim LP, de Stanchina E, Xuan Z, Liang Y, et al. A microRNA component of the p53 tumour suppressor network. Nature. 2007 Jun 28;447(7148):1130-4.

[98] Xu D, Takeshita F, Hino Y, Fukunaga S, Kudo Y, Tamaki A, et al. miR-22 represses cancer progression by inducing cellular senescence. J Cell Biol. 2011 Apr 18;193(2): 409-24.

[99] Levine B, Kroemer G. Autophagy in the pathogenesis of disease. Cell. 2008 Jan 11;132(1):27-42.

[100] Gamerdinger M, Hajieva P, Kaya AM, Wolfrum U, Hartl FU, Behl C. Protein quality control during aging involves recruitment of the macroautophagy pathway by BAG3. Embo J. 2009 Apr 8;28(7):889-901.

[101] Young AR, Narita M, Ferreira M, Kirschner K, Sadaie M, Darot JF, et al. Autophagy mediates the mitotic senescence transition. Genes Dev. 2009 Apr 1;23(7):798-803.

[102] Cosme-Blanco W, Shen MF, Lazar AJ, Pathak S, Lozano G, Multani AS, et al. Telomere dysfunction suppresses spontaneous tumorigenesis in vivo by initiating p53-dependent cellular senescence. EMBO Rep. 2007 May;8(5):497-503.

[103] Feldser DM, Greider CW. Short telomeres limit tumor progression in vivo by inducing senescence. Cancer Cell. 2007 May;11(5):461-9.

[104] Gonzalez-Suarez E, Samper E, Flores JM, Blasco MA. Telomerase-deficient mice with short telomeres are resistant to skin tumorigenesis. Nat Genet. 2000 Sep;26(1):114-7.

[105] Greenberg RA, Chin L, Femino A, Lee KH, Gottlieb GJ, Singer RH, et al. Short dysfunctional telomeres impair tumorigenesis in the INK4a(delta2/3) cancer-prone mouse. Cell. 1999 May 14;97(4):515-25.

[106] Siegl-Cachedenier I, Munoz P, Flores JM, Klatt P, Blasco MA. Deficient mismatch repair improves organismal fitness and survival of mice with dysfunctional telomeres. Genes Dev. 2007 Sep 1;21(17):2234-47.

[107] Akbar AN, Henson SM. Are senescence and exhaustion intertwined or unrelated processes that compromise immunity? Nat Rev Immunol. 2011 Apr;11(4):289-95.

[108] Caruso C, Buffa S, Candore G, Colonna-Romano G, Dunn-Walters D, Kipling D, et al. Mechanisms of immunosenescence. Immun Ageing. 2009;6:10.

[109] Panda A, Arjona A, Sapey E, Bai F, Fikrig E, Montgomery RR, et al. Human innate immunosenescence: causes and consequences for immunity in old age. Trends Immunol. 2009 Jul;30(7):325-33.

[110] Liu Y, Johnson SM, Fedoriw Y, Rogers AB, Yuan H, Krishnamurthy J, et al. Expression of p16(INK4a) prevents cancer and promotes aging in lymphocytes. Blood. 2011 Mar 24;117(12):3257-67.

[111] Menzel O, Migliaccio M, Goldstein DR, Dahoun S, Delorenzi M, Rufer N. Mechanisms regulating the proliferative potential of human CD8+ T lymphocytes overexpressing telomerase. J Immunol. 2006 Sep 15;177(6):3657-68.

[112] Parish ST, Wu JE, Effros RB. Modulation of T lymphocyte replicative senescence via TNF-{alpha} inhibition: role of caspase-3. J Immunol. 2009 Apr 1;182(7):4237-43.

[113] Lynch HE, Goldberg GL, Chidgey A, Van den Brink MR, Boyd R, Sempowski GD. Thymic involution and immune reconstitution. Trends Immunol. 2009 Jul;30(7):366-73.

[114] Larbi A, Dupuis G, Khalil A, Douziech N, Fortin C, Fulop T, Jr. Differential role of lipid rafts in the functions of CD4+ and CD8+ human T lymphocytes with aging. Cell Signal. 2006 Jul;18(7):1017-30.

[115] Fulop T, Kotb R, Fortin CF, Pawelec G, de Angelis F, Larbi A. Potential role of immunosenescence in cancer development. Ann N Y Acad Sci. 2010 Jun;1197:158-65.

[116] Hanahan D, Weinberg RA. Hallmarks of cancer: the next generation. Cell. 2011 Mar 4;144(5):646-74.

[117] Zitvogel L, Tesniere A, Kroemer G. Cancer despite immunosurveillance: immunoselection and immunosubversion. Nat Rev Immunol. 2006 Oct;6(10):715-27.

[118] Campisi J. Cancer and ageing: rival demons? Nat Rev Cancer. 2003 May;3(5):339-49.

[119] Ventura A, Kirsch DG, McLaughlin ME, Tuveson DA, Grimm J, Lintault L, et al. Restoration of p53 function leads to tumour regression in vivo. Nature. 2007 Feb 8;445(7128):661-5.

[120] Xue W, Zender L, Miething C, Dickins RA, Hernando E, Krizhanovsky V, et al. Senescence and tumour clearance is triggered by p53 restoration in murine liver carcinomas. Nature. 2007 Feb 8;445(7128):656-60.

[121] Michaloglou C, Vredeveld LC, Soengas MS, Denoyelle C, Kuilman T, van der Horst CM, et al. BRAFE600-associated senescence-like cell cycle arrest of human naevi. Nature. 2005 Aug 4;436(7051):720-4.

[122] Rakhra K, Bachireddy P, Zabuawala T, Zeiser R, Xu L, Kopelman A, et al. CD4(+) T cells contribute to the remodeling of the microenvironment required for sustained tumor regression upon oncogene inactivation. Cancer Cell. 2010 Nov 16;18(5):485-98.

[123] Reimann M, Lee S, Loddenkemper C, Dorr JR, Tabor V, Aichele P, et al. Tumor stroma-derived TGF-beta limits myc-driven lymphomagenesis via Suv39h1-dependent senescence. Cancer Cell. 2010 Mar 16;17(3):262-72.

[124] Kang TW, Yevsa T, Woller N, Hoenicke L, Wuestefeld T, Dauch D, et al. Senescence surveillance of pre-malignant hepatocytes limits liver cancer development. Nature. 2011 Nov 24;479(7374):547-51.

[125] Hoenicke L, Zender L. Immune surveillance of senescent cells--biological significance in cancer- and non-cancer pathologies. Carcinogenesis. 2011 Nov;33(6):1123-6.

[126] Schreiber RD, Old LJ, Smyth MJ. Cancer immunoediting: integrating immunity's roles in cancer suppression and promotion. Science. 2011 Mar 25;331(6024):1565-70.

Section 5

Mastication and Cognition

Chapter 5

The Relationship Between Mastication and Cognition

Kin-ya Kubo, Huayue Chen and Minoru Onozuka

Additional information is available at the end of the chapter

http://dx.doi.org/10.5772/54911

1. Introduction

Although mastication is primarily involved in food intake and digestion, it also promotes and preserves general health, including cognitive function. Functional magnetic resonance imaging (fMRI) and positron emission topography studies recently revealed that mastication leads to increases in cortical blood flow and activates the somatosensory, supplementary motor, and insular cortices, as well as the striatum, thalamus, and cerebellum [1]. Masticating immediately before performing a cognitive task increases blood oxygen levels (BOLD) in the prefrontal cortex and hippocampus, important structures involved in learning and memory, thereby improving task performance [1]. Thus, mastication may be a drug-free and simple method of attenuating the development of senile dementia and stress-related disorders that are often associated with cognitive dysfunction. Previous epidemiologic studies demonstrated that a decreased number of residual teeth, decreased denture use, and a small maximal biting force are directly related to the development of dementia, further supporting the notion that mastication contributes to maintain cognitive function [2].

Here we provide further evidence supporting the interaction between mastication and learning and memory, focusing on the function of the hippocampus, which is essential for the formation of new memories. We first summarize recent progress in understanding how mastication affects learning and memory. We then describe the impaired function and pathology of the hippocampus in an animal model of reduced mastication using senescence-accelerated prone (SAMP8) mice, and discuss human studies showing that mastication enhances hippocampal-dependent cognitive function. We then describe how occlusal disharmony is a potential chronic stressor that impedes or suppresses hippocampal-mediated learning and memory, suggesting that normal occlusion is essential for producing the ameliorative effects of mastication on stress-induced changes in the hippocampus. Finally, we focus on the ameliorative effects of mastication on stress-induced suppression of learning and memory functions in the hippocampus and on systemic stress responses in both animals and humans.

2. Dysfunctional mastication and cognitive function

Dysfunctional mastication affects cognitive function, and reduced mastication contributes to senile dementia, Alzheimer's disease, and a declining quality of life in the elderly. In particular, the systemic effects of tooth loss are an epidemiologic risk factor for Alzheimer's disease [2]. Missing teeth, due to dental caries and periodontitis are common in the elderly, and reduce their ability to masticate. We created a molarless senescence-accelerated prone (SAMP8) mouse model of dysfunctional mastication by extracting or cutting the upper molar teeth (molarless). SAMP8 mice mature normally for up to 6 months of age, but then exhibit accelerated aging (with a median life span of 12 months compared with 2- to 3 years for other strains). SAMP8 mice show clear aging-related impairments in learning and memory at 6 months of age [3, 4], and these mice are often used in aging studies. Molarless SAMP8 mice exhibit age-dependent deficits in spatial learning in the Morris water maze [5-10] (Fig. 1). The duration of the molarless condition in aged SAMP8 mice correlates with the level of impaired learning [7], and restoring lost molars with artificial crowns attenuates the molarless-induced increases in the learning and memory deficits [9]. Masticatory stimulation is also impaired by a soft-food diet [11], which leads to learning impairment [11]. Together, these findings indicate that masticatory stimulation is closely related to learning and memory.

Several morphologic changes are observed in the hippocampus of molarless mice, including a decreased number of pyramidal cells [6], hypertrophied glial fibrillary acid protein-labeled astrocytes [7, 10] and decreased dendritic spines in the CA1 region [8], suppressed cell proliferation in the dentate gyrus [12]. These behavioral and morphologic changes are very similar to aging-related changes in the hippocampus [13]. The decreased masticatory stimulation resulting from a soft-food diet results in similar morphologic features [14, 15]. Thus, masticatory dysfunction appears to accelerate the aging process in the hippocampus.

Although the relationship between dysfunctional mastication and these behavioral and morphologic changes in the hippocampus is unclear, there are several possible mechanisms.

Decreased mastication decreases the information input from the oral area to the central nervous system, which leads to the degeneration of target cells [16], as exercise promotes axonal sprouting and synaptogenesis [17] and enhances neurogenesis in the hippocampus [18]. Tooth loss or extraction causes degenerative changes in the trigeminal ganglion cell bodies of the primary sensory neurons innervating the teeth [19] and transganglionic degeneration in the secondary neurons in the trigeminal spinal tract nucleus [20]. Hence, the impairment in cognitive function due to masticatory dysfunction might be related to the decreased activity of the sensory pathways of the oral areas. Further, dysfunctional mastication leads to increased decreased cholinergic activity. The number of choline acetyltransferase-positive neurons in

http://dx.doi.org/10.5772/54911

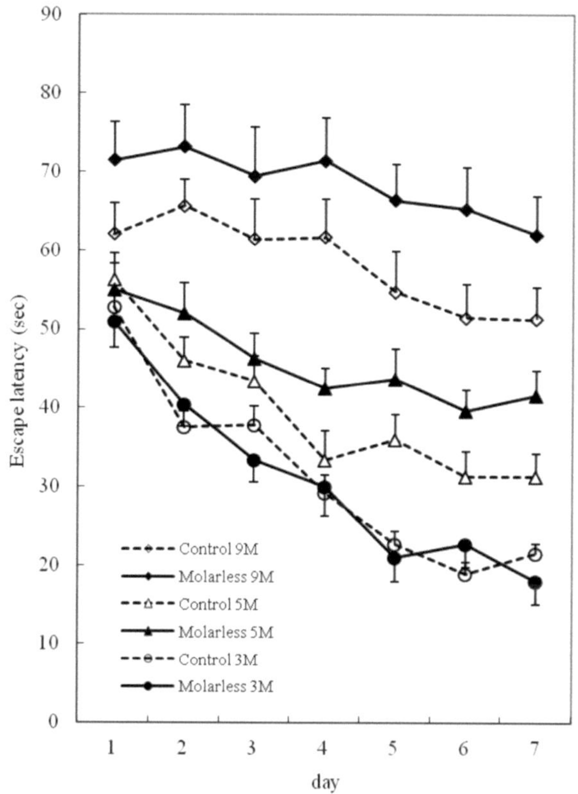

Figure 1. Effect of molarless condition on spatial learning in the Morris water maze test. The results are expressed as the mean score (mean ± SE, n=6 for each group) of four trials per day. Note that 9-month-old molarless mice required a significantly longer time than age-matched controls to reach the platform.

the septal nucleus is decreased in molarless mice [24], and decreased acetylcholine concentrations are observed in the cerebral cortex and hippocampus [24], as well as decreased acetylcholine release [24] in the hippocampus in response to extracellular stimulation. In rodents, spatial memory is associated with acetylcholine levels in the hippocampus [25]. Therefore, the decreased cholinergic activity induced by the molarless condition could contribute learning impairments.

Decreased mastication may also lead to increases in the plasma corticosterone levels. The molarless condition in aged SAMP8 mice increases plasma corticosterone levels [5], and downregulates glucocorticoid receptors (GRs) and GR messenger ribonucleic acid (GR mRNA) in the hippocampus [21]. The hippocampus contains a high density of GR and is involved in the negative feedback mechanism with the hypothalamo-pituitary-adrenal axis via GR, making it very sensitive to corticosterone [22]. The morphologic and behavioral changes in the hippocampus due to chronic stress or long-term exposure to excessive corticosterone are similar to the changes observed with reduced mastication [23]. In support of this notion, treatment with the corticosterone synthesis inhibitor metyrapone prevents molarless-induced learning impairments and neuron loss in the hippocampus [5]. Thus, chronic stress induced by masticatory dysfunction could lead to learning and memory impairments.

Recent fMRI and positron emission tomography studies in humans revealed that several brain regions are activated during mastication [26, 27]. We performed fMRI studies in humans to evaluate the areas of the brain that are activated in association with chewing. In these studies, subjects were asked chew gum with no odor or taste components and perform rhythmic chewing at a rate of approximately 1 Hz. Bilateral increases in activity were observed in several brain areas, including the primary somatosensory cortex, primary motor cortex, supplementary motor area, premotor area, prefrontal cortex, insula, posterior cortex, thalamus, striatum, and cerebellum [26, 27]. Age-dependent changes in the chewing-induced BOLD signals were observed in the primary sensorimotor cortex, cerebellum, and thalamus [26, 27]. The right prefrontal cortex showed the highest increase in activity in elderly persons compared to both young adults and young persons [1] (Fig. 2). The prefrontal cortex is involved in cognitive function [28], and neuronal activity between the right prefrontal cortex and hippocampus might contribute to cognitive function. An fMRI evaluation of the effects of chewing on brain activity during a working memory task showed an increase in BOLD signals in the right premotor cortex, precuneus, thalamus, hippocampus, and inferior parietal lobe [29]. In another fMRI experiment examining the effect of chewing on hippocampal activity in a spatial cognition task [1], subjects were shown 16 photographs followed by the same number of pictures of a plus character (+) on a green background during each cycle. Each picture or photograph was projected every 2 s during the cycle and the subjects were asked to remember as many of the photographs as possible. The hippocampal BOLD signals in young subject were strongly increased but no significant difference was seen before and after chewing, whereas hippocampal activation in aged subject was quite small compared to that in young subject. The activation area and the intensity of the fMRI signals were, however, increased by chewing [1] (Fig. 3 and 4). Memory acquisition in aged subjects is also significantly enhanced by chewing, whereas chewing had no effect in young subject [1] (Fig. 5). These findings in humans support a link between increased hippocampal BOLD signals and enhanced memory acquisition.

Further studies are needed to clarify how the reduced oral input activity to the aging hippocampus resulting from masticatory dysfunction differs from reduced activity of other types sensory pathways.

http://dx.doi.org/10.5772/54911

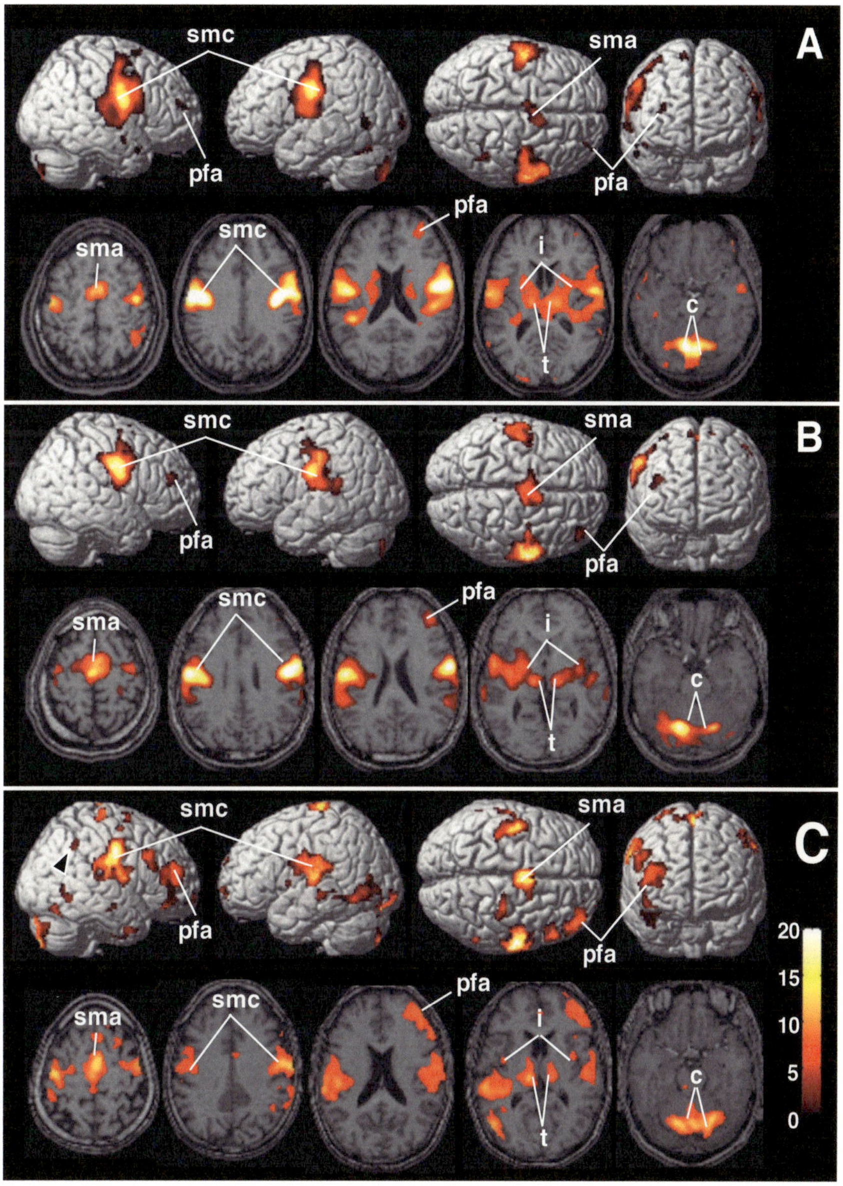

Figure 2. Effects of aging on brain regional activity during chewing. Significant signal increases associated with gum chewing in a young adult subject (A), middle-aged subject (B), and an aged subject (C). Upper section: activated areas superimposed on a template (P<0.05, corrected for multiple comparisons). Lower section: activated regions superimposed on a T1-weighted MRI scan (P<0.01, uncorrected for multiple comparisons). pfa, prefrontal area; sma, supplementary motor area; smc, primary sensorimotor cortex; c, cerebellum; i, insula; t, thalamus. Color scale: t value (degree of freedom=87.12). (Onuzuka et al., 2008, [1] with permission)

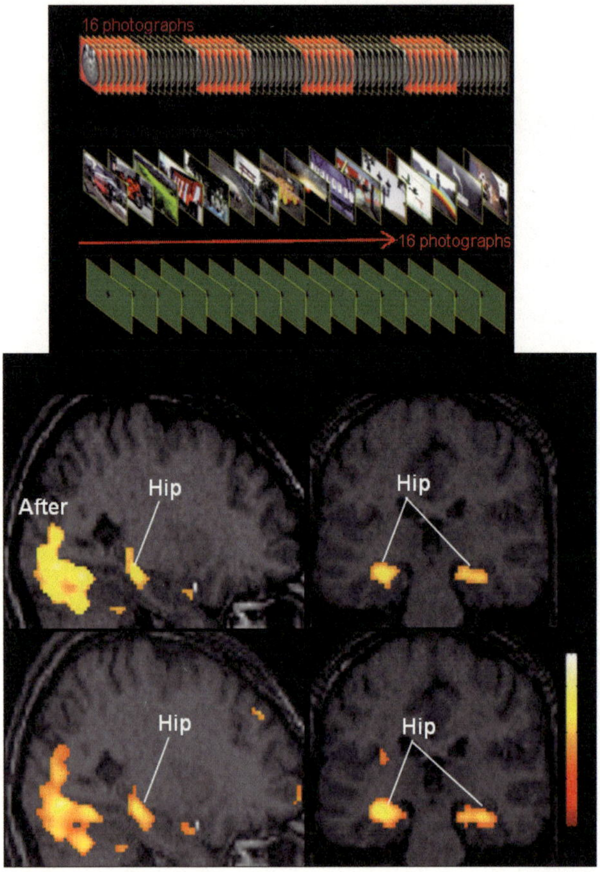

Figure 3. Hippocampal activities in young subject. A Task paradigm. B Significant signal increases associated with photograph encoding before and after gum chewing. Hip, hippocampus. Color scale: t value. (Onozuka et al., 2008, [1] with permission)

3. Occlusal disharmony and cognitive function

Occlusal disharmony, such as loss of teeth and increases in the vertical dimension of crowns, bridges, or dentures, causes bruxism or pain in the masticatory muscles and temporomandibular joints, and general malaise [30, 31]. Studies in SAMP8 mice also show that occlusal disharmony impairs learning and memory. Using SAMP8 mice, we created a model of occlusal disharmony by raising the bite by approximately 0.1 mm using dental materials, referred to as the bite-raised condition. Animals in the bite-raised condition show age-dependent deficits in spatial learning in the Morris water maze [32-39] (Fig. 6). Raising the bite in aged SAMP8 mice decreases the number of pyramidal cells [34] as well as the number of their dendritic spines [39], and increases hypertrophy and hyperplasia of grail fibrillary acid protein-labeled astrocytes [38] in the hippocampal CA1and CA3 regions, suggesting that occlusal disharmony

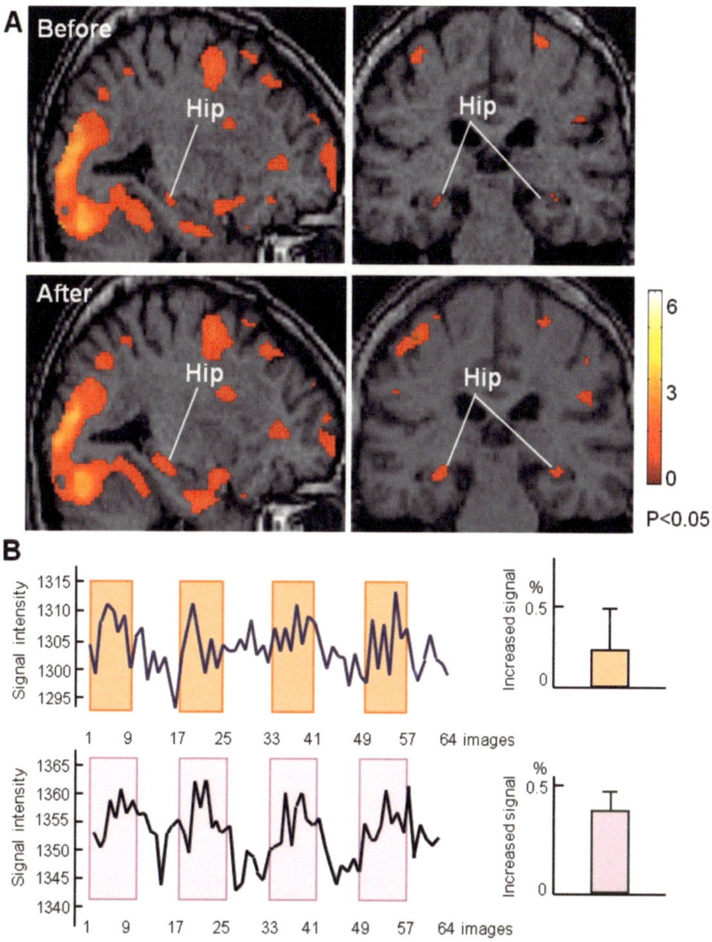

Figure 4. Hippocampal activities in an aged subject. A, Significant signal increases are associated with photograph encoding before and after gum chewing. Color scale: t value. B, Changes in signal intensity on an image-by image basis for 64 successive images during four cycles of encoding of photographs: brown (without chewing) and pink (with chewing) boxes; plus (+) characters (without boxes) (Onozuka et al., 2008, [1], with permission)

resulting from the bite-raised condition also enhances aging-related changes in the hippocampus.

In rodents and monkeys, alterations of the bite alignment induced by attaching acrylic caps to the incisors [40-42] or inserting occlusal splints in the maxilla [43, 44] are associated with increases urinary cortisol levels and plasma corticosterone levels, suggesting that occlusal disharmony is also a source of stress. In support of this notion, aged bite-raised SAMP8 mice with learning deficits exhibit marked increase in plasma corticosterone levels [33, 36, 37] and downregulation of hippocampal GR and GR mRNA [33]. The behavioral and morphologic changes observed in animals with occlusal disharmony closely resemble the changes induced

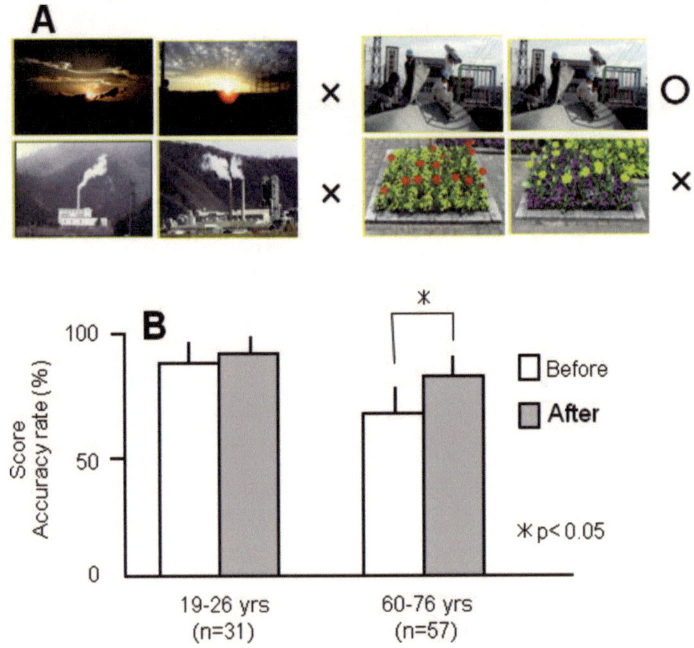

Figure 5. Memory acquisition before and after gum chewing for 2 min. A recall test was carried out 20 min after the encoding experiments. In the recall test, we used 64 photographs at random: 32 of the photographs were repeated from the encoding test, and the other 32 photographs were newly added. The subject had to judge whether each photograph had been seen before. (Onozuka et al., 2008, [1], with permission)

by chronic stress and/or long-term exposure to glucocorticoid exposure [23, 100]. The hippocampus is very sensitive to corticosterone [22]. These hippocampal behavioral and morphologic impairments induced by occlusal disharmony are also attenuated by administration of the corticosterone synthesis inhibitor metyrapone [37]. These findings suggest that occlusal disharmony-induced changes in learning behavioral and hippocampal morphology due to increases in the glucocorticoid levels in association with the downregulation of GR and GR mRNA.

Occlusal disharmony, like masticatory dysfunction, decreases hippocampal activity resulting from the activity of masticatory organ pathways. In bite-raised aged SAMP8 mice, both induction of Fos in the hippocampus following a learning task [36] and the number of spines in hippocampal CA1 pyramidal cells are decreased [39]. Further, the bite-raised condition leads to a decreased number of choline acetyltransferase-positive neurons in the septal nucleus, and reduction in extracellular stimulation-induced acetylcholine release [45].

Occlusal disharmony also affects catecholaminergic activity. Altering the bite by placing an acrylic cap on the lower incisors leads to increases in both dopamine and noradrenaline levels in the hypothalamus and/or frontal cortex [40-42], and decreases in tyrosine hydroxylase, GTP cyclohydroxylase I, and serotonin immunoreactivity in the cerebral cortex, caudate nucleus,

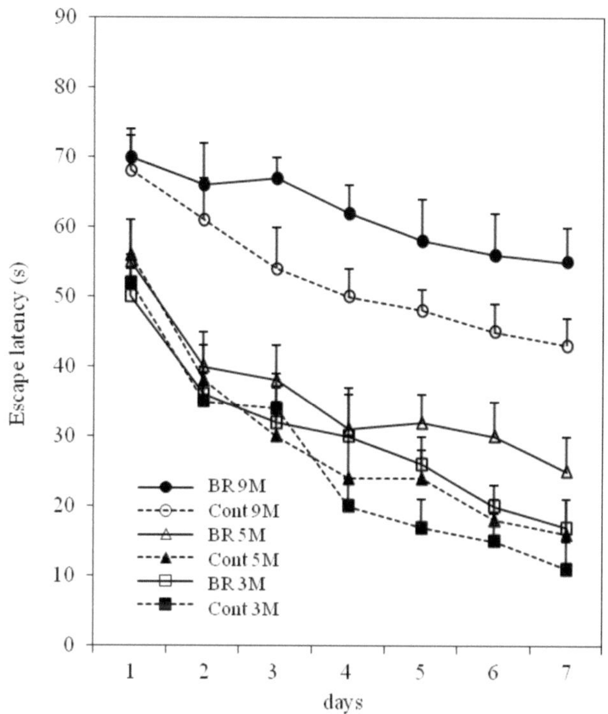

Figure 6. Effect of bite-raised condition on spatial learning in the Morris water maze test. The results are expressed as the mean score (mean ± SE, n=6 for each group) of four trials per day. 9m BR, 9-month-old bite-raised mice; 9m Cont, 9-month-old control mice; 5m BR, 5-month-old bite-raised mice; 5m Cont, 5-month-old control mice; 3m BR, 3-month-old bite-raised mice; 3m Cont, 3-month-old control mice. Note that 9-month-old bite-raised mice required a significantly longer time to reach the platform than age-matched controls. (Kubo et al., 2007, [34])

substantia nigra, locus coeruleus, and nucleus raphe dorsalis [46], which are similar to the changes induced by chronic stress [47]. These changes in the catecholaminergic and serotonergic systems induced by occlusal disharmony likely affect the innervations of the hippocampus. The bite-raised condition impairs neurogenesis and leads to apoptosis in the hippocampal dentate gyrus and decreases the expression of hippocampal brain derived neurotrophic factor, all of which could contribute to the learning impairments observed in animals with occlusal disharmony.

These findings in animal models were extended to humans. In humans, we used a custom-made splint that forced the mandible into a retrusive position and a splint without modification as a control in order to measure BOLD signals during clenching in a malocclusal model [48]. Several regions were activated by clenching, including the premotor cortex, prefrontal cortex, sensorimotor cortex, and insula. In the malocclusion model, which also induces psychologic discomfort, clenching further increased BOLD signals in the anterior cingulate cortex and the amygdala [48]. These findings suggest that clenching under malocclusal conditions induces emotional stress and/or pain-related neuronal processing in the brain.

Together these findings suggest that changes in the hippocampus induced by occlusal disharmony result from increased stress. Occlusal disharmony, like masticatory dysfunction leads to alterations in the central nervous system, especially the hippocampus. Further studies are needed to elucidate differences in the effects of dysfunctional mastication and occlusal disharmony.

4. Mastication and stress coping

The act of chewing, or masticatory stimulation, during stressful conditions may attenuate the effects of stress on cognitive function. To examine the effect of mastication on stress-induced behavioral and morphologic changes, we placed mice in a ventilated plastic restraint tube in which they were only able to move back and forth, but not turn around, to induce restraint stress. Half of mice were given a wooden stick (diameter, ~2mm) to chew during restraint [12]. As mentioned above, the hippocampus plays a crucial role in memory formation and is highly sensitive to aging [49, 50] and stress [51]. Increased plasma corticosterone levels suppress synaptic plasticity in the hippocampus [52] and cell proliferation in the hippocampal dentate gyrus [12] (Fig. 7). Chewing during a stressful event, on the other hand, attenuates stress-induced impairments of plasticity in the hippocampus by activating stress-suppressed N-methyl-D-aspartate-receptor function [53, 54]. Chewing under stress conditions also blocks the stress-induced suppression of cell generation in the hippocampal dentate gyrus [12]. In adults, neurogenesis in the hippocampus is required for hippocampus-dependent learning and memory [55]. Thus, chewing during stress may attenuate stress-induced impairments in cognitive function.

Rodents permitted to chew on a wooden stick during restraint stress showed attenuated restraint-induced increase in plasma corticosterone levels [12] and corticotrophin releasing factor expression [56], c-Fos induction [57], and phosphorylation of extracellular signal-regulated protein kinase 1/2 [58], oxidative stress [59], and nitric oxide [60, 61] in the paraventricular nucleus of the hypothalamus, compared with controls not provided with a wooden stick. Thus, chewing under stressful conditions appears to attenuate stress-induced increase in plasma corticosterone levels by inhibiting the hypothalamo-pituitary-adrenal-axis.

Mastication may also activate histamine neurons through the ventromedial hypothalamus and mesencephalic trigeminal sensory nucleus [62]. The histamine system could modulate the activity of the septohippocampal cholinergic system, which is involved in learning and memory [63]. Chewing under stress conditions increases the release of histamine in the hippocampus by activating H1 receptors [64]. Therefore, chewing may induce changes in the amounts of acetylcholine released, thereby attenuating stress-induced impairments in memory function.

In animals that aggressively chew on a wooden stick during immobilization stress, the stress-induced release of noradrenaline in the amygdala [65] and Fos-immunoreactivity in the right medial prefrontal cortex are increased [66], whereas Fos-immunoreactivity in the right central nucleus of the amygdala [66], and the dopamine response in the medial prefrontal cortex are decreased [67]. The prefrontal cortex has a crucial role in several cognitive, affective, and physiologic processes, and the central nucleus of the amygdala regulates dopamine neurotransmission in the medial prefrontal nucleus [60, 61]. These findings suggest that chewing during stressful conditions modulates catecholaminergic neurotransmission in the central nervous system, leading to changes in cognitive function.

Clinical studies have shown that offspring of mothers who suffer social, emotional or hostile experiences displayed enhanced susceptibility to some mental disorders, including depression, schizophrenia and cognitive deficits [68]. Maternal stress is a suggested risk factor for impaired brain developmental and anxiety, depressive-like behavior and learning deficits in rodents pups [69-71], and maternal stress model is often used in studies for depression and cognitive deficits in pups. We recently evaluated whether chewing during maternal restraint stress prevents stress-induced anxiety-like behavior and learning impairment in pups. Pregnant mice were exposed to restraint stress beginning on day 15 and continuing until delivery. Mice were placed in a ventilated plastic restraint tube in which they were only able to move back and forth, but not turn around, to induce restraint stress. Half of the dams were given a wooden stick (diameter, ~2mm) to chew on during the restraint stress. The pups were raised to adulthood and behavioral and morphologic changes were assessed. Restraint stress during pregnancy caused anxiety-like, impaired learning and suppressed cell proliferation in the hippocampal dentate gyrus. Chewing during restraint stress, however, attenuated the anxiety-like behavior, impaired learning, and suppressed cell generation induced by restraint stress. These findings suggest that maternal chewing contributes to prevent stress-induced anxiety-like behavior, learning impairment, and morphologic changes in hippocampus in pups.

In humans, chewing gum alleviates a negative mood, reduces cortisol levels during acute laboratory-induced psychologic stress [72], and reduces perceived levels of daily stress [73]. These findings indicate that the stress response in human is also ameliorated by chewing.

Additional studies are needed to investigate the mechanisms by which aggressive chewing under stress conditions attenuates stress-induced changes to the brain.

5. Conclusion

Masticatory dysfunction resulting from tooth loss or extraction, feeding on a soft-diet or occlusal disharmony, induces pathologic changes in the hippocampus and deficits in learning and memory. Aggressive biting or chewing activates several regions in the central nervous system, including the right prefrontal cortex, which is strongly involved in learning and memory. Chewing under stressful conditions attenuates stress-induced changes in the brain. These findings together indicate that masticatory function is important for maintaining cognitive function, and chewing during exposure to stress might be a useful method of coping with stress. Chewing gum may thus be a simple method to attenuate or delay the development of dementia and to ameliorate the effects of stress on the brain.

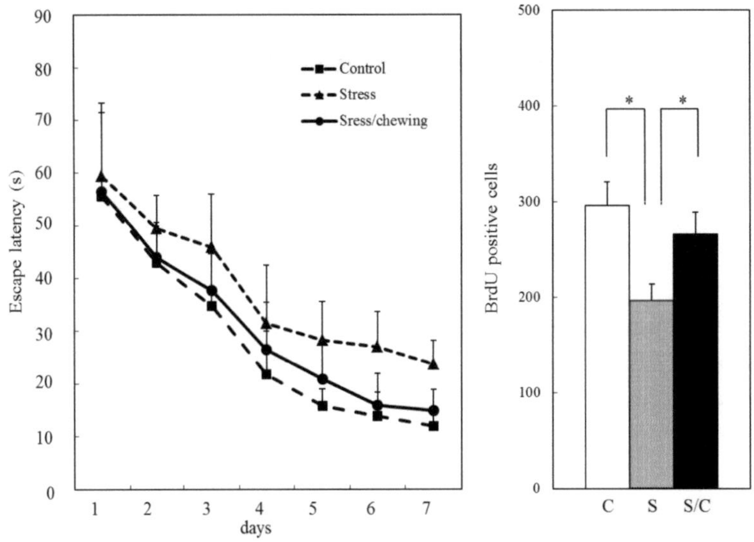

Figure 7. Effect of chewing during prenatal stress on learning ability and cell proliferation in the hippocampal dentate gyrus. Spatial learning in the water maze test (A) and BrdU-positive cells (B). The results are expressed as the mean score (mean ± SD, n=6 for each group) of four trials per day (A). The results are presented as the mean ± SD (n=5 for each group). C, control; S, restraint stress; S/C, restraint/chewing. *$P<0.05$ (B). Note that prenatal stress induced learning and memory deficits, and decreased cell proliferation in the hippocampal dentate gyrus. Maternal chewing during stress inhibits the stress-induced learning and memory deficits, and suppression of cell generation.

Acknowledgements

This work was supported in part by Grant-in Aid Scientific Research from the Ministry of Education, Culture, Sports, Science, and Technology-Japan (KAKENHI 22390395).

Author details

Kin-ya Kubo[1*], Huayue Chen[2] and Minoru Onozuka[3]

*Address all correspondence to: kubo@seijoh-u.ac.jp

1 Seijoh University Graduate School of Health Care Studies, Fukinodai, Tokai, Aichi, Japan

2 Department of Anatomy, Gifu University Graduate School of Medicine, Yanaido, Gifu, Japan

3 Nittai Jusei Medical College for Judo Therapeutics, Yoga, Setagaya-ku, Tokyo, Japan

References

[1] Onozuka M, Hirano Y, Tachibana A, Kim W, Ono Y, Sasaguri K, Kubo K, Niwa M, Kanematsu K, Watanabe K. Interactions between chewing and brain activities in human. In: Onozuka M. and Yen CT. (eds.) Novel Trends in Brain Science Springer; 2008. p 99-113.

[2] Kondo K, Niino M, Shido K. A case-control study of Alzheimer's disease in Japan: significance of life-styles. Dementia 1995; 5(6) 314-326.

[3] Yagi H, Katoh S, Akiguchi I, Takeda T. Age-related deterioration of ability of acquisition in memory and learning in senescence accelerated mouse: SAM-p/8 as an animal model of disturbance in recent memory. Brain Research 1988; 474(1) 86-93.

[4] Flood JF, Morley JE. Learning and memory in the SAMP8 mouse. Neuroscience and Behavioral Reviews 1998; 22(1) 1-20

[5] Onozuka M, Watanabe K, Fujita M, Tonosaki K, Saito S. Evidence for involvement of GC response in the hippocampal changes in aged molarless SAMP8 mice. Behavioral Brain Research 2002; 131(1-2) 125-129.

[6] Onozuka M, Watanabe K, Mirbod SM, Ozono S, Nishiyama K, Karasawa N, Nagatsu I. Reduced mastication stimulates impairment of spatial memory and degeneration of hippocampal neurons in aged SAMP8. Brain Research 1999; 826(1) 148-153.

[7] Onozuka M, Watanabe K, Nagasaki S, Jiang Y, Ozono S, Nishiyama K, Karasawa N, Nagatsu I. Impairment of spatial memory and changes in astroglial responsiveness following loss of molar teeth in aged SAMP8 mice. Behavioral Brain Research 2000; 108(2) 145-155.

[8] Kubo KY, Iwaku F, Watanabe K, Fujita M, Onozuka M. Molarless-induced changes of spines in hippocampal region of SAMP8 mice. Brain Research 2005; 1057(1-2) 191-195.

[9] Watanabe K, Ozono S, Nishiyama K, Saito S, Tonosaki K, Fujita M, Onozuka M. The molarless condition in aged SAMP8 mice attenuates hippocampal Fos induction linked to water maze performance. Behavioral Brain Research 2002; 128(1) 19-25.

[10] Watanabe K, Tonosaki K, Kawase T, Karasawa N, Nagatsu I, Fujita M, Onozuka M. Evidence for involvement of dysfunctional teeth in the senile process in the hippocampus of SAMP8 mice. Experimental Gerontology 2001; 36(2) 283-295.

[11] Yamamoto T, Hirayama A. Effects of soft-diet feeding on synaptic density in the hippocampus and parietal cortex of senescence-accelerated mice. Brain Research 2001; 902(2) 255-263.

[12] Kubo K, Sasaguri K, Ono Y, Yamamoto T, Takahashi T, Watanabe K, Karasawa N, Onozuka M. Chewing under restraint stress inhibits the stress-induced suppression

of cell birth in the dentate gyrus of aged SAM8 mice. Neuroscience Letters 2009; 466 109-113.

[13] deToledo-Morrell L, Geinisman Y, Morrell F. Age-dependent alteration in hippocampal synaptic plasticity: relation to memory disorders. Neurobiology of Aging 1993; 14, 441-446.

[14] Yamamoto T, Hirayama A. Effects of soft-diet feeding on synaptic density in the hippocampus and parietal cortex of senescence-accelerated mice. Brain Research 2001; 902(2) 255-263.

[15] Mitome M, Hasegawa T, Shirakawa T. Mastication influences the survival of newly generated cells in mouse dentate gyrus. Neuroreport 2005; 16(3) 249-252.

[16] Deitch JS, Rubel EW. Rapid changes in ultrastructure during deafferentation-induced atrophy. Journal of Comparative Neurology 1989; 281(2) 234-258.

[17] Chen YC, Chen QS, Lei JL, Wang SL. Physical training modifies the age-related decrease of GAP-43 and synaptophysin in the hippocampal formation in C57BL/6J mouse. Brain Research 1998; 806(2) 238-245.

[18] van Praag H, Kempermann G, Gage FH. Running increases cell proliferation and neurogenesis in the adult mouse dentate gyrus. Nature Neuroscience 1999; 2(3) 266-270.

[19] Kubota K, Nagae K, Shibanai S, Hosaka K, Iseki H, Odagiri N, Lee MS, Chang CM, Ohkubo K, Narita N. Degeneration changes of primary neurons following tooth extraction. Annals of Anatomy 1988; 166(1-5) 133-139.

[20] Gobel S. An electron microscope analysis of the trans-synaptic effects of peripheral nerve injury subsequent to tooth pulp extirpations on neurons in laminae I and II of the medullary dorsal horn. Journal of Neuroscience 1984; 4(9) 2281-2290.

[21] Kubo K, Iwaku F, Arakawa Y, Ichihashi Y, Sato Y, Takahashi T, Watanabe K, Karasawa N, Nagatsu I, Onozuka M. The molarless condition in aged SAMP8 mice reduces hippocampal inhibition of the hypothalamic-pituitary-adrenal axis. Biogenic Amines 2007; 21(6) 309-319.

[22] Meaney MJ, Lupien S. Hippocampus, Overview. In: Fink G. (ed.) Encyclopedia of Stress. Second edition. Academic Press; 2000. p379-386.

[23] Watanabe Y, Gould E, McEwen BS. Stress induces atrophy of apical dendrites of hippocampal CA3 pyramidal neurons. Brain Research 1992; 588(2) 341-345.

[24] Onozuka M, Watanabe K, Fujita M, Tomida M, Ozono S. Changes in the septohippocampal cholinergic system following removal of molar teeth in the aged SAMP8 mouse. Behavioral Brain Research 2002; 133(2) 197-204.

[25] Stancampiano R, Cocco S, Cugusi C, Sarais L, Fadda F. Serotonin and acetylcholine release response in the rat hippocampus during a spatial memory task. Neuroscience 1999; 89(4) 1135-1143.

[26] Onozuka M, Fujita M, Watanabe K, Hirano Y, Niwa M, Nishiyama K, Saito S. Mapping brain region activity during chewing: a functional magnetic resonance imaging study. Journal of Dental Research 2002; 81(11) 743-746.

[27] Onozuka M, Fujita M, Watanabe K, Hirano Y, Niwa M, Nishiyama K, Saito S. Age-related changes in brain regional activity during chewing: a functional magnetic resonance imaging study. Journal of Dental Research 2003; 82(8) 657-660.

[28] Moritz-Gasser S, Duffau H. Cognitive processes and neural basis of language switching: proposal of a new model, Neuroreport 2009; 20(18) 1577-1580.

[29] Hirano Y, Obata T, Kashikura K, Nonaka H, Tachibana A, Ikehira H, Onozuka M. Effects of chewing in working memory processing. Neuroscience Letters 2008; 436 189-192.

[30] Christensen J. Effect of occlusion-raising produces on the chewing system, The Dental Practitioner and Dental Record 1970; 20(7) 61-69.

[31] Umemoto G, Tsukijima Y, Koyano K. The treatment of three patients who insist that indefine complaints arise from occlusion. Japan Journal of Psychosomatic Dentistry 13 1998; 13 133-139. (in Japanese).

[32] Arakawa Y, Ichihashi Y, Iinuma M, Tamura Y, Iwaku F, Kubo KY. Duration-dependent effects of the bite-raised condition on hippocampal function in SAMP8 mice. Okajima Folia Anatomica Japonica 2007; 84(3) 115-119.

[33] Ichihashi Y, Arakawa Y, Iinuma M, Tamura Y, Kubo K, Iwaku F, Sato Y, Onozuka M. Occlusal disharmony attenuates glucocorticoid negative feedback in aged SAMP8 mice. Neuroscience Letters 2007; 427(2) 71-76.

[34] Kubo K, Yamada Y, Iinuma M, Iwaku F, Tamura Y, Watanabe K, Nakamura H, Onozuka M. Occlusal disharmony induces spatial memory impairment and hippocampal neuron degeneration via stress in SAMP8 mice. Neuroscience Letters 2007; 414 188-191.

[35] Iinuma M, Ichihashi Y, Hioki Y, Kurata C, Tamura Y, Kubo K. Malocclusion induces chronic stress. Okajima Folia Anatomica Japonica 2008; 85(1) 35-42.

[36] Kubo K, Ichihashi Y, Iinuma M, Iwaku F, Tamura Y, Karasawa N, Nagatsu I, Onozuka M. Involvement of glucocorticoid response in hippocampal activities in aged SAMP8 mice with occlusal disharmony. Biogenic Amines 2007; 21(5) 273-282.

[37] Kubo K, Iwaku F, Arakawa Y, Ichihashi Y, Iinuma M, Tamura Y, Karasawa N, Nagatsu I, Sasaguri K, Onozuka M. The corticosterone synthesis inhibitor metyrapone

prevents bite-raising induced impairment of hippocampal function in aged senescence-accelerated prone mice (SAMP8). Biogenic Amines 2007; 21(6) 291-300.

[38] Ichihashi Y, Arakawa Y, Iinuma M, Tamura Y, Kubo K, Iwaku F, Takahashi T, Karasawa N, Nagatsu I, Onozuka M. Changes in GFAP-immunoreactive astrocytes induced by the bite-raised condition in aged SAMP8 mice. Biogenic Amines 2008; 22(1-2) 39-48.

[39] Kubo K, Kojo A, Yamamoto T, Onozuka M. The bite-raised condition in aged SAMP8 mice induces dendritic spine changes in the hippocampal region. Neuroscience Letters 2008; 441 141-144.

[40] Areso MP, Giralt MT, Sainz B, Prieto M, Garcĭa-Vallejo P, Gōmez FM. Occlusal disharmonies modulate central catecholaminergic activity in the rat. Journal of Dental Research 1999; 78(6) 1204-1213.

[41] Yoshihara T, Matsumoto Y, Ogura T. Occlusal disharmony affects plasma corticosterone and hypothalamic noradrenaline release in rats. Journal of Dental Research 2001; 80(12) 2089-2092.

[42] Yoshihara T, Taneichi R, Yawaka Y. Occlusal disharmony increases stress response in rats. Neuroscience Letters 2009; 452 181-184.

[43] Budtz-Jørgensen E. A 3-month study in monkeys of occlusal dysfunctional and stress. Scandinavian Journal of Dental Research 1980; 88(3) 171-180.

[44] Budtz-Jørgensen E. Occlusal dysfunction and stress. An experimental study in macaque monkeys. Journal of Oral Rehabilitation 1981; 8(1) 1-9.

[45] Katayama T, Mori D, Miyake H, Fujiwara S, Ono Y, Takahashi T, Onozuka M, Kubo K. Effect of bite-raised condition on the hippocampal cholinergic system of aged SAMP8 mice. Neuroscience Letters, 2012; 520 77-81.

[46] Kubo K, Miyake H, Fujiwara S, Takeuchi T, Hasegawa Y, Toyoda S, Nagatsu I, Ono Y, Yamamoto T, Onozuka M, Karasawa N. Occlusal disharmony reduces catecholaminergic system. Biogenic Amines 2009; 23(1) 9-18.

[47] Feldman S, Weidenfield J. Glucocorticoid receptor antagonists in the hippocampus modify the negative feedback following neural stimuli. Brain Research 1999; 821(1) 33-37.

[48] Otsuka T, Watanabe K, Hirano Y, Kubo K, Miyake S, Sato S, Sasaguri K. Effects of mandible deviation on brain activation during clenching: an fMRI preliminary study. Journal of Craniomandibular Practice 2009; 27(2) 88-93.

[49] Kitraki E, Bozas E, Philippidis H, Stylianopoulou F. Aging-related changes in GF-II and c-foc gene expression in the rat brain. International Jornal of Developmental Neuroscience 1993; 11(1) 1-9.

[50] Olton DS, Becker JT, Handelmann GE. Hippocampus space and memory. Behavioral Brain Science 1979; 2 313-365.

[51] McEwen BS. The neurobiology of stress: from serendipity to clinical relevance. Brain Research 2000; 886(1-2) 172-189.

[52] Kim JJ, Diamond DM. The stressed hippocampus, synaptic plasticity and lost memories. Nature Reviews. Neuroscience 2002; 3(6) 453-462.

[53] Ono Y, Kataoka T, Miyake S, Cheng SJ, Tachibana A, Sasaguri K, Onozuka M. Chewing ameliorates stress-induced suppression of hippocampal long-term potentiation. Neuroscience 2008; 154(4) 1352-1359.

[54] Ono Y, Kataoka T, Miyake S, Sasaguri K, Sato S, Onozuka M. Chewing rescues stress-suppressed hippocampal long-term potentiation via activation of histamine H1 receptor. Neuroscience Research 2009; 64(4) 385-390.

[55] Bruel-Jungerman E, Rampon C, Laroche S. Adult hippocampal neurogenesis, synaptic plasticity and memory: facts and hypothesis. Reviews in the Neuroscience. 2007; 18(2) 93-114.

[56] Hori N, Yuyama N, Tamura K. Biting suppresses stress-induced expression of corticotrophin-releasing factor (CRF) in the rat hypothalamus. Journal of Dental Research 2004; 83(2) 124-128.

[57] Kaneko M, Hori N, Yuyama N, Sasaguri K, Slavicek R, Sato S. Biting suppresses Fos expression in various regions of the rat brain-further evidence that the masticatory organ functions to manage stress. Stomatologie 2004; 101 151-156.

[58] Sasaguri K, Kikuchi M, Yuyama N, Onozuka M, Sato S. Suppression of stress immobilization induced phosphorylation of ERK 1/2 by biting in the rat hypothalamic paraventricular nucleus. Neuroscience Letters 2005; 383(1-2) 160-164.

[59] Miyake S, Sasaguri K, Hori N, Shoji H, Yoshino F, Miyazaki H, Anzai K, Ikota N, Ozawa T, Toyoda M, Sato S, Lee MC. Biting reduces acute stress-induced oxidative stress in the rat hypothalamus. Redox Report; 2005; 19(1) 19-24.

[60] Hori N, Lee MC, Sasaguri K, Ishii H, Kamei M, Kimoto K, Toyoda M, Sato S. Suppression of stress-induced nNOS expression in the rat hypothalamus by biting. Journal of Dental Research 2005; 84(7) 624-628.

[61] Miyake S, Takahashi S, Yoshino F, Todoki K, Sasaguri K, Sato S, Lee MC. Nitric oxide levels in rat hypothalamus are increased by restraint stress and decreased by biting. Redox Report 2008; 13(1) 31-39.

[62] Sakata T, Yoshimatsu H, Masaki T, Tsuda K. Anti-obesity actions of mastication driven by histamine neurons in rats. Experimental Biology and Medicine (Maywood, NJ) 2003; 228(10) 1106-1110.

[63] Mochizuki T, Okakura-Mochizuki K, Horii A, Yamamoto Y, Yamayodani A. Histaminergic modulation of hippocampal acetylcholine release in vivo. Journal of Neurochemistry 1994; 62(6) 2275-2282.

[64] Ono Y, Kataoka T, Miyake S, Sasaguri K, Sato S, Onozuka M. Chewing rescues stress-suppressed hippocampal long-term potentiation via activation of histamine H1receptor. Neuroscience Research 2009; 64(4) 385-390.

[65] Tanaka T, Yoshida M, Yokko H, Tomita M, Tanaka M. Expression of aggression attenuates both stress-induced gastric ulcer formation and increases in noradrenaline release in the rat amygdale assessed by intracerebral microdialysis. Pharmacology, Biochemistry, and Behavior 1998; 59(1) 27-31.

[66] Stalnaker TA, España RA, Berridge CW. Coping behavior causes asymmetric changes in neuronal activation in the prefrontal cortex and amygdale. Synapse 2009; 63(1) 82-85.

[67] Berridge CW, Mitton E, Clark W, Roth RH. Engagement in a non-escape (displacement) behavior elicits a selective and lateralized suppression of frontal cortical dopaminergic utilization in stress. Synapse 1999; 32(3) 187-197.

[68] O'Connor TG, Heron J, Golding J, Glover V. Maternal antenatal anxiety and behavioural/emotional problem in children: a test of a programming hypothesis. Journal of Child Psychology and Psychiatry 2003; 44 1025-1036.

[69] Lemaire V, Koehl M, Le Moal M, Abrous N. Prenatal stress produces learning deficits associated with an inhibition of neurogenesis in the hippocampus. Proceeding of the National Academy of Science of the United States of America 2000; 97(20) 11032-11037.

[70] Mohammad HS, Hossein H. Prenatal stress induces learning deficits and is associated with a decrease in granules and CA3 cell dendritic tree size in rat hippocampus. Anatomical Science International 2007; 82 21-217.

[71] Weinstock M. The long-term behavioural consequences of prenatal stress. Neuroscience and Biobahavioral Reviews 2008; 32(6) 1073-1086.

[72] Scholey A, Haskell C, Robertson B, Kennedy D, Miline A, Wetherell M. Chewing gum alleviates negative mood and rescues cortisol during acute laboratory psychological stress. Physiology and Behavior 2009; 97(3-4) 304-312.

[73] Zibell S, Madansky E. Impact of gum chewing on stress levels: online self-perception research study. Current Medical Research and Opinion 2009; 25(6) 1491-1500.

Section 6

Neurodegenerative Disease

Chapter 6

On the Way to Longevity: How to Combat Neuro-Degenerative Disease

Patrizia d'Alessio, Rita Ostan, Miriam Capri and Claudio Franceschi

Additional information is available at the end of the chapter

http://dx.doi.org/10.5772/54914

1. Introduction

1.1. Aging and inflammaging

Aging can be defined as the accumulation of unrepaired, deleterious changes occurring in the molecules, cells, tissues and organs of the body over time generated by internal and external sources. An integral part of the aging process is represented by the adaptive mechanisms that the body sets up to compensate and neutralize the adverse effects of such damage that lead to a progressive change of the body composition and its microenvironments. Among others, the multifaceted dynamic process, known as immunosenescence, encompasses all the complex changes occurring in the immune system during aging. It results from the adaptation process of the body to the continuous challenge of infections and is the basis of the age-associated decrease in immune competence that renders individuals more susceptible to diseases. Immunosenescence is associated with an increase of morbidity and mortality [27, 35, 46]. One of the typical aspects of immunosenescence is the profound modification within the cytokine network leading to the development of a low-grade inflammatory status, known as "inflammaging" [28]. This phenomenon is characterized by a general increase in plasmatic levels and cell capability to produce pro-inflammatory cytokines (Interleukin-6, IL-6, Interleukin-1, IL-1 and Tumour Necrosis Factor-α, TNF-α) and by a subsequent increase of the main inflammatory markers, such as C-reactive protein (CRP) and serum amyloid A (A-SAA) [29, 31, 32]. This generalized pro-inflammatory status, interacting with the genetic background and environmental factors, potentially triggers the onset of the most important age-related diseases, such as cardiovascular diseases, atherosclerosis, metabolic syndrome, type 2 diabetes and obesity, neurodegeneration, arthrosis and arthritis, osteoporosis and osteoarthritis, sarcopenia, major depression and frailty [46]. The first evidence of the age-associated modification in the balance of cytokine network was described by [24] who found an increase of IL-6 plasma levels and a corresponding decrease of IL-2 production in healthy elderly subjects [24, 26].

We have provided several contributions on the relevance of the inflammatory reaction at the vascular site for cell senescence in terms of the reversibility of its inflammatory phenotype [16, 17]. These data could be confirmed by *ex vivo* data of Franceschi's laboratory. A significant increase of IL-6, TNF-α and IL-1β levels were described in mitogen-stimulated cultures from aged donors. Indeed, cells from aged people seem able to up-regulate the production of these cytokines in response to appropriate stimuli indicating that the cellular machinery for the production of these molecules remains active and efficient during aging [24]. It has been hypothesized that inflammaging could be due to the antigenic load and its persistence for the entire lifespan. Antigens of common viruses such as human cytomegalovirus (HCMV) or Epstein-Barr virus (EBV) represent a major driving force for the activation of macrophages and expansion of specific T cell clones (megaclones) producing a large amount of inflammatory cytokines [54, 55]. The increase with age of IL-6 plasma levels appears to be unexpectedly present in both those who underwent successful aging and those who suffered pathological aging. Thus, we must question the factors responsible for successful aging. Data obtained on centenarians by the Franceschi laboratory showed that centenarians also are inflamed [3, 4, 26]. Thus, inflammaging *per se* is not incompatible with longevity. But it is likely that many protective factors, such as the genetic background, epigenetic markers [33] and anti-inflammatory molecules can play a pivotal role in counteracting unfavourable pro-inflammatory signalling [32].

At present it is not understood whether the alteration in the regulation of inflammatory reactions could be a cause or rather an effect (or both in a vicious cycle) of the aging process as a whole. A wide range of elements has been claimed to contribute to the development of low-grade inflammation. In particular, in addition to the main impact of the immune system, a variety of tissues (adipose tissue and muscle in particular), organs (liver and brain) and ecosystems (skin, mouth, vagina and gut microbiota) differently contribute to inflammaging onset, progression and persistence having specific organ-restricted and/or systemic effects [13].

Gut microbiota and the gastrointestinal-associated immune system coexist in a balanced microenvironment where cytokines and lymphocytes have to cope with the antigenic load, in order to control the enormous variety of bacterial species within the intestinal microflora. During aging, subtle changes in intestinal microbial structure may contribute to the age-related inflammatory status. A reduction of some populations of *Clostridia* in favour of enrichment in facultative anaerobes in centenarians has been described. In addition, the remodelling of centenarians' microbiota was associated with an increased inflammatory state, determined by a series of peripheral inflammatory markers (IL-6, IL-8) [7]. The dysbiosis observed in these extremely long-lived subjects represents an important source of continuous antigenic stimulation (immune/inflammatory/toxic/metabolic) to other organs and systems, such as the immune system and the liver, contributing to the development and maintenance of inflammaging. So why are healthy centenarians the best example of successful ageing, even if they are characterized by inflammaging? Our hypothesis is that their reduced capacity to mount strong inflammatory responses is due to a remarkable genetic pattern (based on anti-inflammatory gene variants) and is able to limit the inflammatory process. A protective genetic component towards the development of age-related pathologies with a strong inflammatory pathogenesis would thus be exerted [32].

Inflammaging can, in turn, undermine the balance between gut microbiota and the gastrointestinal-associated immune system, contributing to the establishment of a vicious inflammatory cycle [8]. Importantly, recent literature suggests the impact of microbiota inflammatory stimuli on the brain [6]. Several studies even suggest an inflammatory pathogenesis at the basis of activation of microglia in response to injury, illness and aging, as described in the following section.

2. Neuro-inflammation

The term neuro-inflammation designates chronic, CNS-specific, inflammation-like glial responses that do not reproduce the classic characteristics of inflammation in the periphery but that may provoke neuro-degenerative events, including plaque formation, dystrophic neurite growth and unwarranted tau phosphorylation, among other signs. Aetiology of neuro-inflammation is not yet clarified even if many strides forward have been made in this field. In fact, during the last decades important discoveries have been made, particularly on risk factors, genetic-associated variants, pro-inflammatory molecules, cellular and sub-cellular modified processes and, ultimately, the gene expression pathways shared in many neuro-degenerative diseases, such as AD. A recent review summarizes microarray human studies in neuro-degenerative diseases showing gene expression profiles shared in these age-associated diseases [15], highlighting the inflammatory component. In addition, RNA splicing and protein turnover are found to be disrupted and mitochondrial dysfunction has been reported.

Franceschi's team is heavily involved in the study of age-related diseases and in particular AD, either in terms of nuclear and mitochondrial genetic variants and pro-inflammatory environments [21, 22, 36-39, 45, 49]. It is well known that AD is a fast growing worldwide pathology: it is a slowly progressive and, after early stage reversible phases, irreversible neuro-degenerative disease. Patients undergo decades of symptomatic progression; multiple interacting molecular mechanisms contribute to the development of the early clinical prodromal stages characterized by episodic memory deficits and decline, as well as impairment of general cognitive functioning, particularly during the final syndromal dementia stage (reviewed in [34]). In the context of AD research, the team studied the role of genetic cytokines variants, such as IL-1, IL-6, TNF-α and interferon-gamma (IFN-γ), in AD patients. The data showed the association between the plasmatic and brain level of IL-6 and IL-6 polymorphisms at 174 position in the promoter region, suggesting a relationship between specific gene variants and circulating levels of a specific inflammatory cytokine; furthermore, cytokine blood level mirrors the quantity of its level in the brain [38]. Similarly, increased levels of IL-1, another pro-inflammatory cytokine, are observed in association with specific IL-1 gene variants [21]. We think that these findings can be integrated into the more general vision of the inflammaging process, i.e. the chronic age-related pro-inflammatory status together with unfavourable genetic variants can contribute to neuro-inflammation pathogenesis and the onset of AD or neuro-degenerative diseases [30, 11]. Many inflammatory mediators have been detected in regions of the brain of patients with AD [45] according to the hypothesis that inflammation might contribute to the neuro-degeneration characterizing this pathology [42].

The activation of the microglia may be due either to local and/or systemic inflammation. In fact, a strong local inflammatory stimulus, such as a previous head trauma, is a risk factor for AD onset and several epidemiological studies clearly show that blood elevations of acute phase proteins, markers of systemic inflammatory stimuli, may be risk factors for cognitive decline and dementia [21, 52]. Moreover, in AD, astrocytes are involved in the production of neurotoxic substances, such as reactive oxygen and nitrogen species, pro-inflammatory cytokines, complement proteins, and other inflammatory mediators that bring about important neuro-degenerative changes [53].

However, the scenario is much more complex than previously thought. The Franceschi group also identified key molecular actors, such as proteasome and immune-proteasome (the molecular complex induced by INFs), as possible motors of protein turnover alteration [43]. The immune-proteasome has been associated with neuro-degenerative and autoimmune diseases as a marker and regulator of inflammatory mechanisms. Its expression in the brain may occur upon neuro-inflammation in different cell types and affect a variety of homeostatic and inflammatory pathways including the oxidized protein clearance and the self-antigen presentation. Recently, its role in epilepsy has been established. In fact the pathology-specific pattern of immune-proteasome expression could provide insight into the complex neuro-inflammatory pathogenic components of this disease [44]. The same group is currently working on the circulating proteasome/immuneproteasome, in order to establish its role as a possible early-biomarker in neuro-degenerative and inflammatory diseases. In this regard, the circulating mitochondrial DNA, another systemic biomarker of inflammation and disease, is also being investigated [57]. This type of research could be strategic for the improvement of therapeutic intervention, one of the priorities of the current European and US research. The possibility, as well as the difficulty, of identifying a pro-inflammatory prodromal phenotype which will develop the syndromic stage, is crucial for the prevention, diagnosis and therapy of AD and other age-related neuro-degenerative pathologies [56].

The study of post-operative delirium (POD) in elderly patients [1, 2] has been promoted by the same approach. Recent literature suggests the presence of an inflammatory component in the POD onset, showing again the close relationship between systemic inflammation and CNS, particularly when a stressful event such as surgery (or anaesthesia) or infectious diseases may provoke an acute exacerbation (delirium) interacting with pre-intra and post-operative parameters. One of the main hypotheses related to the delirium onset is that peripherally produced pro-inflammatory cytokines enter the brain and activate microglia. Activated microglia may produce inflammatory mediators affecting neuronal functioning, that may be implicated in the symptomatology of delirium.

What are the physiological mechanisms to counteract the pro-inflammatory activation of neuro-inflammation? One of the best characterized is the cholinergic inhibition that controls microglia activation and thereby limits the severity and duration of delirium. If cholinergic inhibition fails, either because of pre-existing neuro-degeneration or use of drugs with anticholinergic effects, neuro-inflammation could spin out of control, leading to severe prolonged delirium that can become associated with dementia [51]. Thus, the first event, i.e., POD, is often a prodromal event for the development of dementia or AD, i.e., a long-term cognitive decline and also an increased mortality. On this last point limited literature is currently available. It is noteworthy that the inflammatory markers are already abundantly present before the post-operative delirium episode (in particular IL-6, IL-8 and CRP) [5] and sometimes this pro-inflammatory status is accompanied by the decrease of anti-inflammatory molecules such as Acetylcholinesterase enzyme (AchE), inducing an imbalance between pro- and anti-inflammatory responses [12].

In progress data from the Franceschi laboratory suggest that the assessing of the level of specific plasmatic pro-inflammatory cytokines, together with other parameters [2], before surgery could be the best strategy for early identification of patients who could develop POD and not only for the best management of patients on the ward. This could lead to fast tracking of elderly patients who could develop neuro-degenerative diseases in the future.

Another model studied by the same laboratory is Down Syndrome (DS), a progeroid syndrome characterized by an accelerated neuro-degenerative process [25, 40]. Ongoing analyses on a cross sectional cohort by means of an ad hoc test battery for cognitive and functional assessments could be essential in gathering evidence on brain areas that first undergo neuro-degeneration.

The strategy for counteracting these different age-related neuro-degenerative clinical pictures and diseases is of primary importance and represents one of most fascinating areas in the field of aging and age-related disease research. In order to slow down and counteract the "destiny" of early identified risk factors in an elderly patient candidate for surgical treatment, what could be the most eligible non-invasive and non-toxic therapeutic intervention? Our driving hypothesis is that we can restrain the onset and the progression of the age-related neuro-degenerative diseases counteracting immunosenescence [10] and inflammaging by diet intervention, moderate and daily physical exercise and the possible use of natural compounds, whose formulation allows specifically reducing inflammatory markers in tissues, cells and blood.

3. Anti-inflammaging/anti-stress intervention

Chronic inflammation is an underlying cause of many apparently unrelated, age-related diseases. This fact is often overlooked, yet persuasive scientific evidence exists that correcting a chronic inflammatory disorder will enable many of the infirmities of aging to be prevented or reversed. When we envisage a link between aging and recurrent or chronic inflammation, we refer to the pathological consequences of inflammation in well-documented medical literature. Regrettably, the origins as well as the consequences of systemic inflammation continue to be an unsolved problem. By following specific prevention protocols (such as weight loss), the inflammatory stimulation could be significantly reduced. An important role in preventing the onset of a chronic inflammatory condition has been attributed either to the practice of a physical activity or to the prescription of a personalized diet, or both.

Terpens are a large and varied class of organic components classified as secondary metabolites. They are produced by a wide variety of plants, particularly conifers, though also by some insects, such as swallowtail butterflies, which emit terpens from their osmeterium. They are the major components of resin and of turpentine produced from resin. The name terpen is derived from the word "turpentine". The smaller and more volatile terpenoids (C10 and C15) are generally the main constituents of the essential oils obtained from many types of plants and flowers, widely used as natural flavourings for food, as fragrances in perfumes in aromatherapy and in traditional and alternative medicines. Terpenoids possess a common structural feature: they contain an integral number of C5 units (isoprene-like) giving a basic molecular formula (C5H8)n for the hydrocarbons series. They are derived from the metabolism of acetate by the mevalonic acid branch biosynthetic pathways of plants.

Examples of monoterpens (C10) are geraniol and limonene. In particular, *d*-limonene has a pronounced chemotherapeutic activity and minimal toxicity in pre-clinical studies. A phase I clinical trial performed to assess toxicity, maximum tolerated dose (MTD) and pharmacokinetics in patients with advanced cancer was followed by a limited phase II evaluation in breast cancer. We have previously published some *in vitro* results on a tri-terpen [58], implicating a NF-κB dependent anti-inflammatory mechanism of action of the extract of *Trytergium Wolfordii* hoek, used in traditional Chinese medicine for the prevention of arthritis, rheumatoid arthritis and arthrosis.

In performing the experiments for the assessment of the doses to be administered in an *in vivo* rodent model, an anti-stress effect of the terpen AISA 5203-L was unexpectedly revealed by a functional observation battery (FOB). A plethora of parameters addressing behavioural, physiological and neurological parameters in female rats submitted to several stressful conditions were measured. Results showed important effects leading to the capacity of the animals to tolerate stress and even pain when compared to vehicle-treated animals [9].

To these preliminary pre-clinical data we were recently able to add some clinical data showing the coherence of our anti-inflammatory/anti-stress approach [18, 19]. The European Capacity study "Ristomed" enrolled 125 healthy individuals from three different countries (Italy, France and Germany). They all received an 'optimal diet for the elderly' with the supplementation of some nutraceutic compounds for a period of 56 days. The diet was developed on the basis of the current recommendations for elderly people and personalized individual dietary requirements, with particular attention given to food compounds that can affect inflammation, oxidative stress and gut microbiota, such as polyunsaturated fatty acids (PUFAs), antioxidant vitamins, polyphenols, flavonoids and fibres. The diet was adapted to the dietary habits for each country. AISA Therapeutics treatment (here referred to as OPE, i.e., Orange Peel Extract) associated as dietary supplementation in addition to the Ristomed diet was validated as an anti-inflammatory food complement.

In this article, we will report the results concerning the inflammatory markers and the (concomitant) alterations of the mood, comparing the group receiving the diet without supplementation (14 males, mean age 69.6 ± 4.1 years; 17 females, 71.3 ± 3.8 years) to that receiving a diet supplemented with daily soft gel capsules containing the terpen extract AISA 5203-L (14 males, mean age 70.6 ± 4.4 years; 16 females, 69.6 ± 3.3 years), related to as OPE (Orange Peel Extract).

The laboratory measurements performed included erythrocyte sedimentation rate (ESR), high-sensitivity C-reactive protein (CRP), white blood cell count (WBC) and fibrinogen measurements. Baseline plasma levels of ESR, CRP, WBC, fibrinogen, IL-6 and TNF-α were used to calculate an inflammation score. This enabled the separation of the patients into two groups of respectively low and high inflammation, so that inflammatory status could be evaluated according to the scores of these markers.

Moreover, several self-assessment questionnaires were analysed to investigate quality of life parameters. The SF-36v2 Health Survey was used to evaluate what each subject felt about his/her health using 36 items covering functional status, wellbeing and an overall evaluation of health, that together are referred to as Quality of Life (QoL). Two summary scores — Physical Component Summary (PCS) and Mental Component Summary (MCS) — were calculated to distinguish a possible physical dysfunction and bodily pain from psychological distress and emotional problems. The State-Trait Anxiety Inventory-X (STAI-X) questionnaire was used to assess the anxiety state and trait, and to describe each subject's feelings at a particular point.

The results of this investigation showed that among clinically healthy, aged subjects (i.e., absence of cancer, obesity, metabolic syndrome, diabetes, major cardiovascular complaints, arthritis or dementia), a third of them showed important inflammatory markers' expression. It is precisely these patients that could be at risk of developing delirium in the case of surgical treatment [2]. They would largely be advantaged by a preventive treatment of their inflammatory condition, especially if high levels of IL-6 and TNF-α are measured.

Conclusively, the results confirmed the anti-inflammatory action of the terpen extract in an aged matched (65-85) healthy population (figure 1 and [20], www.ristomed.eu).

Moreover, Ristomed results were conclusive also for the capacity to lower anxiety and thus implicitly for the link between inflammation and anxiety. Interestingly, study results obtained for quality of life assessment (PCS, MCS and GHQ-12), mood (STAI-X) and depression (CES-D) confirmed our findings on mood modulation. We note in particular that OPE treatment was more effective in high-inflamed patients, the anti-depressive effect is more visible in low-inflamed patients (figure 2). These results also confirm previous findings established by our Functional Observation Battery (FOB) in rodents, where AISA 5203-L supplementation was able to substantially contribute to pain tolerance and mood stabilization. However, the most intriguing result was the fact that the stressed animal (non-pathological stress stimulating anxiety), instead of developing a freezing attitude, following oral administration of the food supplement, developed an activity. These data can be useful to answer the question "Is stress relevant for cell senescence and thus aging?". The important effects on mood in the presence of stress situations has been documented for decades. The mechanism by which a stress is responsible for detrimental organ impairment seems to reside in the complex interconnections between inflammatory and immunosenescence pathways [14, 23, 41, 50].

In conclusion, inflammaging is an age-related process arising from the interaction with the genetic/epigenetic/microbioma–specific background and the environment, as shown in figure 3, and this interaction potentially triggers the onset of the most important age-related diseases. In this regard, lessons from the clinical research teach us that inflammation as well as mood alterations seem relevant for the onset of degenerative diseases. The balancing between pro- and anti-inflammatory agents can be modified by external stimuli both in terms of stress or

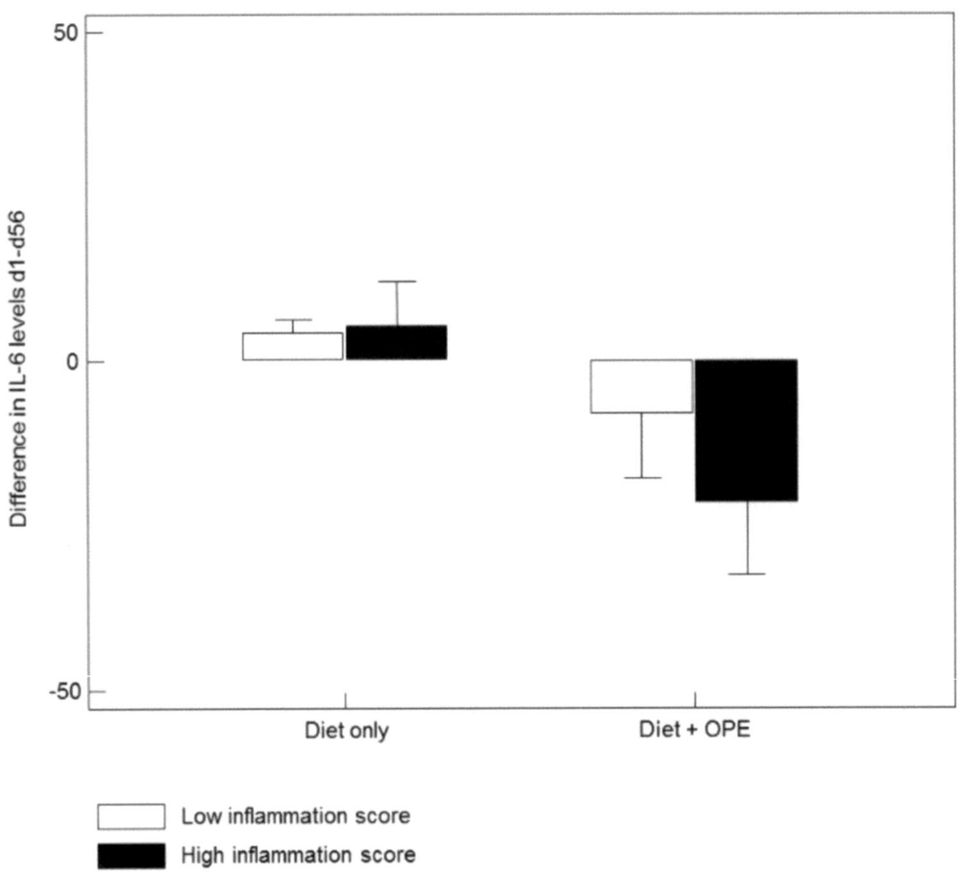

Figure 1. Results of the Ristomed study: inflammation sub-groups and IL-6 variation in diet versus diet plus terpen extract AISA 5203-L, in the figure mentioned as OPE (i.e., Orange Peel Extract).

anti-stress effects. The evidence that post-surgery delirium episodes precipitating dementia are announced by anxiety that in turn is associated to high inflammatory scores, allows us to research efficacious presides to treat these cases. A preventive administration of non-toxic food additives counteracting inflammation and soothing mood alterations could be integrated into the daily diet preceding the surgical intervention. A preventive administration of highly anti-inflammatory specific biocomplements should be included in the recommendations to the healthy aged population by medical institutions and supported by healthy aging guidelines in western countries.

Finally, in order to counteract inflammatory stimuli and to modulate the impact of the environment on inflammaging, we proposed to intervene with diet and food supplementation.

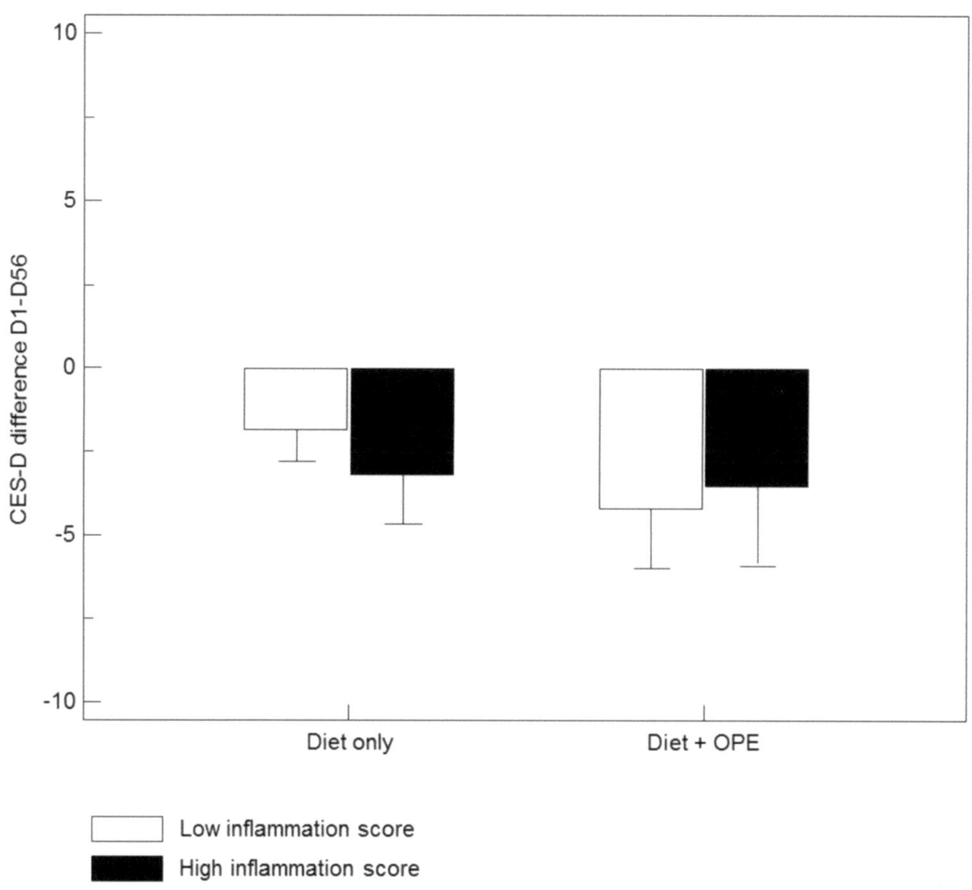

Figure 2. Inflammation subgroups and CES-D variation in diet versus diet plus OPE.

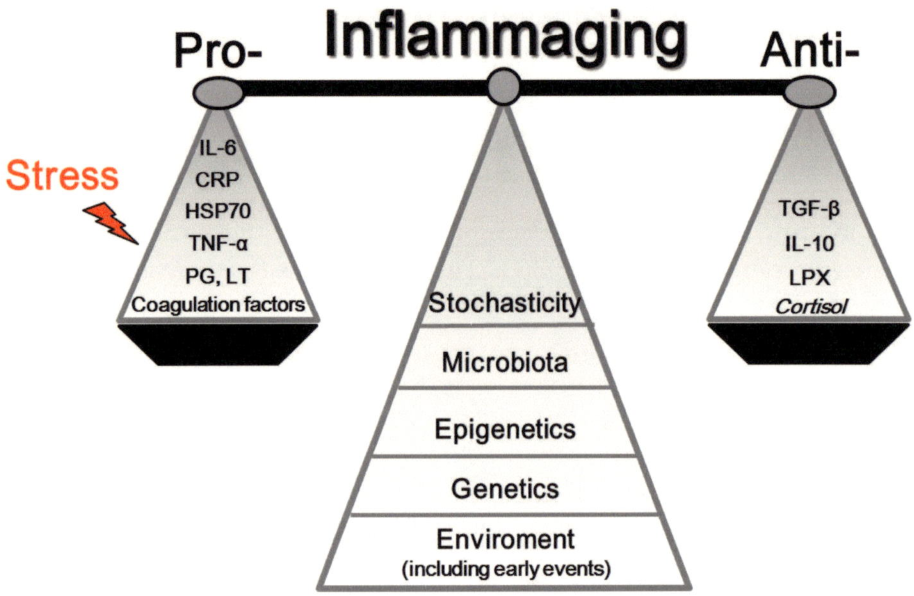

Figure 3. The Inflammaging balance. The low, chronic pro-inflammatory status, characterizing aging interacts with genetic/epigenetic/microbiota background and potentially triggers the onset of the most important age-related diseases. The balancing between pro- and anti-inflammatory agents can be modified by external stimuli, such as stress or anti-stress (diet and anti-inflammatory compounds). PG: prostaglandins; LT: leukotrienes, LPX: lipoxins

Author details

Patrizia d'Alessio[1], Rita Ostan[2], Miriam Capri[2] and Claudio Franceschi[2]

1 University Paris Sud-11 and Biopark Cancer Campus 1, Villejuif, France

2 Department of Experimental, Diagnostic and Specialty Medicine, University of Bologna, Italy

References

[1] Agnoletti V, Ansaloni L, Catena F, Chattat R, De Cataldis A, Di Nino G, Franceschi C, Gagliardi S, Melotti RM, Potalivo A, Taffurelli M. Postoperative Delirium after elective and emergency surgery: analysis and checking of risk factors. A study protocol. BMC Surg. 2005 5:12.

[2] Ansaloni L, Catena F, Chattat R, Fortuna,D, Franceschi C, Mascitti P, Melotti R M. Risk factors and incidence of postoperative delirium in elderly patients after elective and emergency surgery. Br J Surg. 2010 97(2):273-80.

[3] Baggio G, Donazzan S, Monti D, Mari D, Martini S, Gabelli C, Dalla Vestra M, Previato L, Guido M, Pigozzo S, Cortella I, Crepaldi G, Franceschi C. Lipoprotein(a) and lipoprotein profile in healthy centenarians: a reappraisal of vascular risk factors. FASEB J (1998). 12, 433–437.

[4] Barbieri M, Ferrucci L, Ragno E, Corsi A, Bandinelli S, Bonafè M, Olivieri F, Giovagnetti S, Franceschi C, Guralnik J M, Paolisso G. Chronic inflammation and the effect of IGF-I on muscle strength and power in older persons. Am J Physiol Endocrinol Metab. 2003 284(3):E481-7.

[5] Beloosesky Y, Hendel D, Weiss A, Hershkovitz A, Grinblat J, Pirotsky A, Barak V. Cytokines and C-reactive protein production in hip-fracture-operated elderly patients. J Gerontol A Biol Sci Med Sci. 2007 62(4):420-6.

[6] Berer K, Mues M, Koutrolos M, Rasbi Z A, Boziki M, Johner C, Wekerle H, Krishnamoorthy G. Commensal microbiota and myelin autoantigen cooperate to trigger autoimmune demyelination. Nature. 2011 479(7374):538-41.

[7] Biagi E, Nylund L, Candela M, Ostan R, Bucci L, Pini E, Nikkilä J, Monti D, Satokari R, Franceschi, C, Brigidi, P, & De Vos, W. Through ageing, and beyond: gut microbiota and inflammatory status in seniors and centenarians. PLoS One. (2010) 5(5):e10667. Erratum in: PLoS One. 2010;5(6).

[8] Biagi E, Candela M, Fairweather-tait S, Franceschi C, Brigidi P. Aging of the human metaorganism: the microbial counterpart. Age (Dordr). 2012 34(1):247-67.

[9] Bisson JF, Menut C, d'Alessio P. New pharmaceutical interventions in aging. Rejuvenation Research. 2008; Vol. 11, No. 2: 399-407.

[10] Capri M, Monti D, Salvioli S, Lescai F, Pierini M, Altilia S, Sevini F, Valensin S, Ostan R, Bucci L, Franceschi C. Complexity of anti-immunosenescence strategies in humans. Artif Organs. (2006).;30(10):730-42.

[11] Caruso C, Franceschi C, Licastro F. Genetics of neurodegenerative disorders. N Engl J Med. (2003).;349(2):193-4.

[12] Cerejeira J, Nogueira V, Luís P, Vaz-serra A, Mukaetova-ladinska E B. The cholinergic system and inflammation: common pathways in delirium pathophysiology. J Am Geriatr Soc. (2012).; 60(4):669-75.

[13] Cevenini E, Caruso C, Candore G, Capri M, Nuzzo D, Duro G, Rizzo C, Colonna-Romano G, Lio D, Di Carlo D, Palmas MG, Scurti M, Pini E, Franceschi C, Vasto S. Age-related inflammation: the contribution of different organs, tissues and systems. How to face it for therapeutic approaches. Curr Pharm Des. (2010). 16(6), 609-618(10)

[14] Chandola T, Britton A, Brunner E, Hemingway H, Malik M, Kumari M, Badrick E, Kivimaki M, Marmot M. Work stress and coronary heart disease: what are the mechanisms? Eur Heart J. (2008).

[15] Cooper-Knock J, Kirby J, Ferraiuolo L, Heath P R, Rattray M, Shaw P J. Gene expression profiling in human neurodegenerative disease. Nat Rev Neurol. 2012 8(9), 518-30.

[16] d'Alessio P, Endothelium as pharmacological target. Curr Op Invest Drugs. 2002; Vol 2, No. 12:1720-1724.

[17] d'Alessio P. Aging and the endothelium. Exp Gerontol. 2004; 39(2):165-171.

[18] d'Alessio P. New Anti-Inflammatory Molecule AISA 5203-L promotes adaptive strategies in cell aging. in: Adaptation Biology and Medicine, Cell Adaptations and Challenges, eds. Wang P, Kuo CH, Takeda N, Singal PK. Narosa Publishing House Ltd. 2011 Vol 6: 369-378.

[19] d'Alessio P, Bennaceur-Griscelli A, Ostan R and Franceschi C. New Targets for the Identification of an Anti-Inflammatory Anti-Senescence Activity. in: Senescence, ISBN 978-953-308-28-6 In-Tech open access. 2012 chap.2: 647-666.

[20] d'Alessio P, Ostan R, Valentini L, Bourdel-Marchasson I, Pinto A, Buccolini F, Franceschi C, Bené MC. Gender differences in response to dietary supplementation by Orange Peel Extract in elderly people in the RISTOMED study: impact on Quality of Life and inflammation. PRIME. 2012 July/August:30-37.

[21] Di Bona Di Plaia A, Vasto S, Cavallone L, Lescai F, Franceschi C, Licastro F, Colonna-Romano G, Lio D, Candore G, Caruso C. Association between the interleukin-1β polymorphisms and Alzheimer's disease: a systematic review and meta-analysis. Brain Res Rev. (2008). 59(1), 155-63.

[22] Di Bona D, Candore G, Franceschi C, Licastro F, Colonna-Romano G, Cammà C, Lio D, Caruso C. Systematic review by meta-analyses on the possible role of TNF-α polymorphisms in association with Alzheimer's disease. Brain Res Rev. (2009). 61(2), 60-8.

[23] Esler M, Eikelis N, Schlaich M, Lambert G, Alvarenga M, Kaye D, Osta A, Guo L, Barton D, Pier C, Brenchley C, Dawood T, Jennings G, Lambert E. Human sympathetic nerve biology: parallel influences of stress and epigenetics in essential hypertension and panic disorder. Ann NY Acad Sci. (2008). 1148, 338-48.

[24] Fagiolo U, Cossarizza A, Scala E, Fanales-Belasio E, Ortolani C, Cozz, E, Monti D, Franceschi C, Paganelli R. Increased cytokine production in mononuclear cells of healthy elderly people. Eur J Immunol (1993). 23(9), 2315-2378.

[25] Franceschi C, Monti D, Scarfí M R, Zeni O, Temperani P, Emilia G, Sansoni P, Lioi M B, Troiano L, Agnesini C et al. Genomic instability and aging. Studies in centenarians (successful aging) and in patients with Down Syndrome (accelerated aging). Ann N Y Acad Sci. (1992). 663, 4-16.

[26] Franceschi C, Monti D, Sansoni P, Cossarizza A. The immunology of exceptional individuals: the lesson of centenarians. Immunol Today (1995). 16(1), 12-16.

[27] Franceschi C, Passeri M, De Benedictis G, Motta L. Immunosenescence. Aging (Milano) 1998 10: 153–154.

[28] Franceschi C, Bonafè M, Valensin S, Olivieri F, De Luca M, Ottaviani E, De Benedictis G. Inflammaging. An evolutionary perspective on immunosenescence. Ann N Y Acad Sci. 2000 Jun;908:244-54.

[29] Franceschi C, Valensin S, Bonafè M, Paolisso G, Yashin A. I, Monti D, De Benedictis G. The network and the remodeling theories of aging: historical background and new perspectives. Exp Gerontol. 2000; 35: 879–896.

[30] Franceschi C, Valensin S, Lescai F, Olivieri F, Licastro F, Grimaldi L. M, Monti D, De Benedictis G, Bonafè M. Neuroinflammation and the genetics of Alzheimer's disease: the search for a pro-inflammatory phenotype. Aging (Milano). (2001).;13(3):163-70.

[31] Franceschi C, Capri M, Monti D, Giunta S, Olivieri F, Sevini F, Panourgia M P, Invidia L, Celani L, Scurti M, Cevenini E, Castellani G C, Salvioli S. Inflammaging and anti-inflammaging: a systemic perspective on aging and longevity emerged from studies in humans. Mech Ageing Dev. (2007). 128(1), 92-105.

[32] Franceschi C. Inflammaging as a major characteristic of old people: can it be prevented or cured? Nutr Rev. 2007 65: S173-6.

[33] Gentilini D, Mari D, Castaldi D, Remondini D, Ogliari G, Ostan R, Bucci L, Sirchia S M, Tabano S, Cavagnini F, Monti D, Franceschi C, Di Blasio A M, Vitale G. Role of epigenetics in human aging and longevity: genome-wide DNA methylation profile in centenarians and centenarians' offspring. Age (August 2012).

[34] Hampel H, Prvulovic D, Teipel S, Jessen F, Luckhaus,C, Frölich L, Riepe M W, Dodel R, Leyhe T, Bertram L, Hoffmann W, Faltraco F. German Task Force on Alzheimer's Disease (GTF-AD). The future of Alzheimer's disease: the next 10 years. Prog Neurobiol. (2011). 95(4), 718-28.

[35] Larbi A, Franceschi C, Mazzatti D, Solana R, Wikby A, Pawelec G. Aging of the immune system as a prognostic factor for human longevity. Physiology (Bethesda). (2008). 23, 64-74.

[36] Lescai F, Pirazzini C, Agostino D, Santoro G, Ghidoni A, Benussi R, Galimberti L, Federica D, Marchegiani E, Cardelli F, Olivieri M, Nacmias F, Sorbi B, Bagnoli S, Tagliavini S, Albani F, Martinelli D, Boneschi,F, Binetti G, Forloni G, Quadri P, Scarpini E, Franceschi C. Failure to replicate an association of rs5984894 SNP in the PCDH11X gene in a collection of 1,222 Alzheimer's disease affected patients. J Alzheimer's Dis. (2010). 385-8.

[37] Lescai F, Chiamenti A M, Codemo A, Pirazzini C, Agostino D, Ruaro G, Ghidoni C, Benussi R, Galimberti L, Esposito D, Marchegiani F, Cardelli F, Olivieri M, Nacmias F,

Sorbi B, Tagliavini S, Albani F, Martinelli D, Boneschi F, Binetti G, Santoro A, Forloni G, Scarpini E, Crepaldi G, Gabelli C, Franceschi C. An APOE haplotype associated with decreased ε4 expression increases the risk of late onset Alzheimer's disease. J Alzheimers Dis. (2011). 24(2), 235-45.

[38] Licastro F, Grimaldi L M, Bonafè M, Martina C, Olivieri F, Cavallone L, Giovanietti S, Masliah E, Franceschi C Interleukin-6 gene alleles affect the risk of Alzheimer's disease and levels of the cytokine in blood and brain. Neurobiol Aging. (2003).24(7):921-6.

[39] Listì F, Candore G, Balistreri C R, Grimaldi M P, Orlando V, Vasto S, Colonna-Romano G, Lio D, Licastro F, Franceschi C, Caruso,C. Association between the HLA-A2 allele and Alzheimer disease. Rejuvenation Res. (2006). 9(1), 99-101.

[40] Lockrow JP, Fortress AM, Granholm AC. Age-related neurodegeneration and memory loss in Down Syndrome. Curr Gerontol Geriatr Res. 2012 463909.

[41] McGeer EG, McGeer PL. The importance of inflammatory mechanisms in Alzheimer disease. Exp Gerontol. 1998 Aug;33(5):371-8.

[42] May L, van den Biggelaar A H, van Bodegom D, Meij H J, de Craen A J, Amankwa J, Frölich M, Kuningas M, Westendorp R G. Adverse environmental conditions influence age-related innate immune responsiveness. Immun Ageing. 2009 30:6-7.

[43] Mishto, M, Bellavista, E, Santoro, A, Stolzing, A, Ligorio, C, Nacmias, B, Spazzafumo, L, Chiappelli M, Licastro F, Sorbi S, Pession A, Ohm T, Grune T, Franceschi C. Immunoproteasome and LMP2 polymorphism in aged and Alzheimer's disease brains. Neurobiol Aging. (2006). Jan;, 27(1), 54-66.

[44] Mishto M, Ligorio C, Bellavista E, Martucci M, Santoro A, Giulioni M, Marucci G, Franceschi C. Immunoproteasome expression is induced in mesial temporal lobe epilepsy. Biochem Biophys Res Commun. (2011). 408(1), 65-70.

[45] Mrak R E, Sheng J G, Griffin W S. Glial cytokines in Alzheimer's disease: review and pathogenic implications. Hum Pathol. (1995). 26(8), 816-23.

[46] Ostan R, Bucci L, Capri M, Salvioli S, Scurti M, Pini E, Monti D, Franceschi C. Immunosenescence and immunogenetics of human longevity. Neuroimmunomodulation. (2008). 15(4-6), 224-240.

[47] Passeri G, Pini G, Troiano L, Vescovini R, Sansoni P, Passeri M, Gueresi P, Delsignore R, Pedrazzoni M, Franceschi C. Low vitamin D status, high bone turnover, and bone fractures in centenarians. J Clin Endocrinol Metab. (2003). 88(11),5109-15.

[48] Santoro A, Balbi V, Balducci E, Pirazzini C, Rosini F, Tavano F, Achilli A, Siviero P, Minicuci N, Bellavista E, Mishto M, Salvioli S, Marchegiani F, Cardelli M, Olivieri F, Nacmias B, Chiamenti A M, Benussi L, Ghidoni R, Rose G, Gabelli C, Binetti G, Sorbi S, Crepaldi G, Passarino G, Torroni A, Franceschi C. Evidence for sub-haplogroup h5 of mitochondrial DNA as a risk factor for late onset Alzheimer's disease. PLoS One. (2010). 5(8):e12037.

[49] Scola L, Licastro F, Chiappelli M, Franceschi C, Grimaldi L M, Crivello A, Romano G, Candore,G, Lio D, Caruso C. Allele frequencies of +874T -A single nucleotide polymorphism at the first intron of IFN-gamma gene in Alzheimer's disease patients. Aging Clin Exp Res. (2003). 15(4), 292-5.

[50] Shibeshi W A, Young-Xu,Y, Blatt C M. Anxiety worsens prognosis in patients with coronary artery disease.J Am Coll Cardiol. (2007). 49(20)

[51] Van Gool W A, van de Beek D, Eikelenboom P Systemic infection and delirium: when cytokines and acetylcholine collide. Lancet. (2010). 375(9716), 773-5.

[52] Vasto S, Candore G, Duro G, Lio D, Grimaldi M P, Caruso C. Alzheimer's disease and genetics of inflammation: a pharmacogenomic vision. Pharmacogenomics. 2007; 8: 1735-45.

[53] Vasto S, Candore G, Listì F, Balistreri C R, Colonna-Romano G, Malavolta M, Lio D, Nuzzo D, Mocchegiani E, Di Bona D, Caruso C. Inflammation, genes and zinc in Alzheimer's disease. Brain Res Rev. (2008). 58(1), 96-105.

[54] Vescovini R, Biasini C, Fagnoni F F, Telera A R, Zanlari L, Pedrazzoni M, Bucci L, Monti D, Medici M C, Chezzi C, Franceschi C, Sansoni P. Massive load of functional effector CD4+ and CD8+ T cells against cytomegalovirus in very old subjects. Journal of Immunology (Baltimore, Md: 1950). 2007; 179 (6):4283-4291.

[55] Vescovini R, Biasini C, Telera A R, Basaglia M, Stella A, Magalini F, Bucci L, Monti D, Lazzarotto T, Dal Monte P, Pedrazzoni M, Medici M C, Chezzi C, Franceschi C, Fagnoni FF, Sansoni P. Intense antiextracellular adaptive immune response to human cytomegalovirus in very old subjects with impaired health and cognitive and functional status. Journal of Immunology (Baltimore, Md: 1950) 2010:184 (6):3242-3249.

[56] Weksler M E, Pawelec G, Franceschi C. Immune therapy for age-related diseases.Trends Immunol. (2009). 30(7), 344-50.

[57] Zhang Q, Raoof M, Chen Y, Sumi,Y, Sursal T, Junger W, Brohi K, Itagaki K, Hauser C J. Circulating mitochondrial DAMPs cause inflammatory responses to injury. Nature. 2010 Mar 4;464(7285):104-7.

[58] Zhang DH, Marconi A, Xu LM, Yang CX, Sun GW, Feng XL, Xu SM, Ling CQ, Qin WZ, Uzan G, and d'Alessio P. Tripterine, inhibits the expression of adhesion molecules in activated endothelial cells. Journ Leuko Biol. 2006; vol 80:309-319.